Sex Research and
Sex Therapy

Routledge Advances in Sociology

Sex Research and Sex Therapy

A Sociological Analysis of Masters and Johnson

Ross Morrow

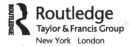

Routledge
Taylor & Francis Group
New York   London

Routledge
Taylor & Francis Group
711 Third Avenue
New York, NY 10017

Routledge
Taylor & Francis Group
2 Park Square
Milton Park, Abingdon
Oxon OX14 4RN

© 2008 by Ross Morrow
Routledge is an imprint of Taylor & Francis Group, an Informa business

First issued in paperback 2012

ISBN13: 978-0-415-40652-9 (hbk)
ISBN13: 978-0-415-54215-9 (pbk)

Library of Congress Cataloging-in-Publication Data

Morrow, Ross, 1962-
    Sex research and sex therapy : a sociological analysis of Masters and Johnson / Ross Morrow.
        p. ; cm. -- (Routledge advances in sociology ; 32)
    Includes bibliographical references and index.
    ISBN 978-0-415-40652-9
    1. Masters, William H. Human sexual response. 2. Masters, William H. Human sexual inadequacy. 3. Johnson, Virginia E. 4. Sex (Biology)--Research--United States--History--20th century. 5. Sex therapy--Research--United States--History--20th century. 6. Sexology--Research--United States--History--20th century. 7. Sex (Biology)--Social aspects--United States. 8. Sex therapy--Social aspects--United States. 9. Sexology--Social aspects--United States. I. Title. II. Series.
    [DNLM: 1. Masters, William H. Human sexual response. 2. Masters, William H. Human sexual inadequacy. 3. Johnson, Virginia E. 4. Sexology. 5. Research Design. 6. Sexual Behavior. 7. Sexual Dysfunction, Physiological. 8. Sexual Dysfunctions, Psychological. HQ 21 M883s 2007]

QP251.M67 2007
612.6072--dc22
                                                                    2007009902

Visit the Taylor & Francis Web site at
http://www.taylorandfrancis.com

and the Routledge Web site at
http://www.routledge.com

Contents

Contents

Acknowledgments

Most of the research for this book occurred while I was working at the University of Newcastle, New South Wales. This was during a time of substantial decline in relative public funding of Australian universities despite healthy federal budget surpluses. This decline of funding was compounded by the well-publicised financial difficulties of the university itself. The declining funds and the resulting squeeze on academic labour, not surprisingly, led to many adverse consequences, including the loss of time for research, reflection and writing. This undoubtedly delayed the research for this book which was not completed until I left the university in 2005. Given the difficult gestation of the research, I am particularly grateful to those people who kindly helped and supported me during this time.

Rachel Sharp has been a wonderful mentor, friend and supporter who believed in this project all the way through and who kindly gave me assistance whenever I needed it. She was particularly helpful with some of the more difficult issues that came up. Mervyn Hartwig and Caroline New both made helpful comments on an earlier version of the manuscript. They, along with Rachel, have been most supportive colleagues and friends. Together, they also exposed me to an engaging and stimulating intellectual milieu outside my university environment. This has enlivened my interests and imagination, deepened my knowledge and sharpened my critical skills.

My friend and colleague Peter Khoury has been an unfailing source of support, encouragement, good ideas and sagely advice. He also read and gave valuable feedback on key parts of the manuscript. Without his kind assistance this book would not have been produced and I owe him more than I can say here. Robert Irvine generously and frequently passed on references and research material he came across while trawling through the research literature. He was a supportive friend and colleague and a critical interlocutor with me about many issues. Karen McLeod gave patient, cheerful and invaluable assistance in typing, formatting and revising the original manuscript.

My late friend and colleague Dennis McIntyre was an enthusiastic supporter of my work. He was a true friend over many years and through difficult and challenging times. He is greatly missed and I am very sad that he did not live to see this work completed. I would especially like to thank my parents—John and Marion Morrow—for their generous and continuing support, help and encouragement over many decades. Their very kind assistance has been crucial to me finishing the research and preparing it for publication. I would also like to thank *Revue Sexologique/The Sexological Review* for kind permission to include material in chapters five and six from a previously published article 'A critique of Masters' and Johnson's concept and classification of sexual dysfunction'. This was originally published in *Revue Sexologique/Sexological Review* (1996) vol. 4, no. 2, pages 159–180. Finally, I would like to thank Routledge for believing in this work and for backing it. Without their invaluable support and input this monograph might never have been produced. Needless to say, I take responsibility for the final contents.

R M

ABOUT THE AUTHOR

Ross Morrow has a PhD in sociology and has published nationally and internationally in the fields of sociology, social theory and human sexuality. He currently teaches social theory at the University of Sydney and social science at the University of Technology, Sydney.

1 Introduction

This book is intended as a contribution to the sociology of sex. It is primarily concerned with William Masters and Virginia Johnson's (1966; 1970) scientific sex research and its clinical applications within the field of sex therapy. Masters (1915–2001) was a U.S. obstetrician and gynecologist, and Johnson (1925–) was his research assistant and later co-researcher. Together, they were two of the most significant and influential sexologists of the twentieth century (Dein 1993/1994; Strong 1993). They are generally regarded as the most important researchers to have scientifically studied human sexual functioning and they are widely acclaimed as the founders of sex therapy in the latter half of the twentieth century. They are internationally renowned, their books have been best sellers, and they have been honoured with more than a dozen awards each from professional groups for their contributions to the scientific study of sex. Their scientific work was also an important exemplar of 'essentialism', in a particularly strong form. Essentialism is the most dominant and influential paradigm in sex research (Masters, Johnson and Kolodny 1985; Weeks 1985; Bullough 1994d; Harding 1998, 12).

The major aim of this book is to provide a sociological analysis and critique of the conceptual foundations and practice of Masters and Johnson's (1966; 1970) sex research and therapy, as articulated in their 'seminal' texts *Human Sexual Response* and *Human Sexual Inadequacy*. The kind of critique offered here is primarily an 'internal' critique of the main themes and ideas in these books. However, I also explore some of the wider theoretical, conceptual and historical issues pertaining to the sociology of sex. These include a discussion of the major theoretical perspectives on human sexuality, and a recuperation of the forgotten history of the sociology of sex. A key theme in my overall argument is that Masters and Johnson constructed their apparently scientific ideas about sexual function and dysfunction with reference to dominant Western beliefs and values about sexuality, and that their sex therapy program operated as an institution of social control.

The book does not attempt to make a comprehensive sociological study of all Masters and Johnson's work. Nor does it claim to offer a 'sociology of knowledge' of their work. Apart from an internal critique of their

1

project, such research would arguably need to address a range of other pertinent issues, including a sociological account of sex therapy as a profession; the history, organisation and internal workings of Masters and Johnson's research institute; a study of the social processes and practices through which they produced and disseminated their 'knowledge'; an examination of their workshops, training sessions, media exposure and annual conferences; an analysis of their entire corpus of published and unpublished works, including their more popular writings; their professional relationships with other sexologists; and their personal relationships with each other, including their marriage, divorce and retirement, and Masters' illness and eventual death from Parkinson's disease. This kind of wider study might also usefully examine the relationship between the sex therapy industry initiated by Masters and Johnson in 1970, and the wider therapeutic, medical and individualising culture of the United States which has been analysed in the work of authors such as Sennett (1977), Lasch (1980), Zilbergeld (1983), Hewitt (1998) and Conrad (2005).

I have primarily focused my attention on the study and analysis of *Human Sexual Response* and *Human Sexual Inadequacy* for three main reasons. Firstly, these two books are probably Masters and Johnson's most original, robust, famous and influential works. *Human Sexual Response* reported on a sex research project which aimed, for the first time, to produce definitive scientific information about human sexual physiology. It involved the largest ever direct laboratory study of human sexual response in 694 men and women over an eleven-year period from 1954 to 1965. In reporting the 'definitive' findings of their research, Masters and Johnson (1966) argued that the sexual responses of males and females are so similar that they can be understood as occurring within a single four stage human sexual response cycle. The model of this cycle formed the centrepiece of their book.

With the publication of *Human Sexual Response*, Masters and Johnson became world famous almost overnight. Their research attracted international media attention and their book became a best seller (Brecher 1970, 28; Belliveau and Richter 1971, 59). Their research findings were largely accepted as scientific fact even though some critics disapproved of their research methods (Belliveau and Richter 1971, 64; Gagnon 1975, 137). Medical schools across the United States began using Masters and Johnson's text to teach new courses on human sexual response and their model of the human sexual response cycle was incorporated (with some amendments) into the American Psychiatric Association's (1980) *Diagnostic and Statistical Manual of Mental Disorders (DSM-III)*. It was used as a model of normal human sexual functioning ('Playboy Interview: Masters and Johnson' 1976, 131, 162; American Psychiatric Association 1980).

Human Sexual Inadequacy achieved its fame and influence for a number of different reasons. Firstly, it provided what was probably the first new system for classifying sexual dysfunctions since the Middle Ages (Boyle

1994, 108). It became the prototype for the sexological diagnosis of sexual dysfunctions after 1970, and its categories of sexual dysfunction were incorporated into the *DSM-III* (1980) as official mental disorders (Irvine 1990a, 192-3). Furthermore, Masters and Johnson themselves continued to rely heavily on this system of classification for many years after it was first formulated (Masters et al 1985; 1994). Secondly, *Human Sexual Inadequacy* contained 'new' ideas about the aetiology of sexual dysfunctions. In contrast to the previously dominant psychoanalytic view that sexual dysfunctions were caused by deep unconscious conflicts, Masters and Johnson (1970) put forward the view that sexual dysfunctions were predominantly caused by fear of sexual inadequacy, and excessive self-monitoring (the adoption of a 'spectator role') during sexual activity. Thirdly, Masters and Johnson introduced a 'new' approach to the treatment of sexual dysfunctions. This involved a rapid, intensive, treatment program, treatment of couples by male and female cotherapists (such as a doctor and psychologist), and the integration of specific therapeutic strategies into an overall treatment package. Fourthly, Masters and Johnson provided an unprecedented report on the effectiveness of their sex therapy program. They reported the results of treating 790 patients for sexual dysfunctions over an eleven year period from January 1959 to December 1969. This is still the largest study of treatment outcomes for sexual dysfunction which has ever been reported (Heiman and Meston 1997, 149). In addition, the study provided follow-up data on patients five years after they had first been treated in order to indicate how many had reverted to a sexually dysfunctional state. Masters and Johnson reported that their new sex therapy program was highly successful with an overall failure rate of only 20%. This failure rate seemed incredibly low in comparison to psychoanalysis which was the main form of treatment for sexual dysfunctions prior to Masters and Johnson.

The publication of *Human Sexual Inadequacy* was greeted with widespread celebration, acclaim and optimism that sexual dysfunctions 'could be substantially eliminated' before the end of the decade (Zilbergeld and Evans 1980, 30). There was very little critical analysis of Masters and Johnson's (1970) claims (Zilbergeld and Evans 1980). Their book, and the work on which it reported, made a major contribution to the development of sex therapy as a new type of specialist occupation. An estimated 5,000 sex therapy clinics developed across the United States in the wake of publication of *Human Sexual Inadequacy*, and sex therapists soon developed their own certifying organisations and professional journals (Heidenry 1997, 172; Zilbergeld and Evans 1980, 30). Sex therapy has developed, and been modified, since the publication of *Human Sexual Inadequacy*, but Masters and Johnson's treatment approach still forms the basis of most sex therapy programs (Bancroft 1986, 172; Davison and Neale 1994, 379; Wiederman 1998, 89; Everaerd 2001; Goren 2003, 495).

The second reason for primarily focusing my attention on *Human Sexual Response* and *Human Sexual Inadequacy* is that these two books, and the projects they describe, cannot be adequately understood in isolation from each other. These two books provide accounts of two integral and inter-related components of what is almost a single overarching research and clinical program. This program sought to describe and understand normal human sexual response partly in order to help understand the causes, types and treatment of sexual dysfunctions. The research and clinical programs discussed in these books were not only closely connected by their rationales. They also substantially overlapped and ran in parallel. For example, Masters and Johnson's research on sexual physiology ran from 1954 to 1965 while their clinical program for the treatment of sexual dysfunction ran from 1959 to 1970. The findings of these two programs also had reciprocal influences on each other. For example, Masters and Johnson's model of the human sexual response cycle was later used as a norm of healthy sexual functioning in their clinical treatment program. Similarly, when research participants had problems with their sexual performances during the labo-ratory research, Masters and Johnson drew on their clinical experiences to assist these participants to develop more 'successful' sexual responses.

Thirdly, it is quite surprising that, despite the apparently momentous scientific, therapeutic and cultural significance of Masters and Johnson's (1966; 1970) work, there has been a marked lack of critical attention to it, including by sociologists. To my knowledge, no large scale systematic soci-ological study of this work has previously been undertaken, completed or published. Nor has there been any extended and detailed sociological anal-ysis of the main arguments and ideas put forth in *Human Sexual Response* and *Human Sexual Inadequacy*. The small number of books which are concerned with Masters and Johnson's (1966; 1970) research and therapy are primarily non-sociological, and expository, serving mainly to introduce and explain this work to a general audience (see, for example, the books by Brecher and Brecher 1968; Belliveau and Richter 1971; and Lehrman 1976). As discussed in chapter 2, there is a small sociological literature on Masters and Johnson's laboratory research and therapy program. This mainly consists of book chapters and journal articles (and even sections of chapters and articles) most of which are not primarily concerned with Mas-ters and Johnson. This literature is also relatively fragmented, and focused on selective and partial aspects of their work. In addition, this literature has often been non-cumulative. Researchers have been unable to build on previous studies because they have not been aware of them. Consequently, one of the main aims of this study is to combine original analysis of Mas-ters and Johnson's (1966; 1970) work, with the findings of the existing literature, in order to develop a more systematic account and evaluation of their project.

My research approach relies on a broadly 'social constructionist' theo-retical perspective. It is primarily used to analyse the rationale, process and outcomes of Masters and Johnson's research and therapy programs in rela-tion to various social factors which affected their work. In particular, this approach is used to analyse and criticise Masters and Johnson's unsubstantiated and strongly essentialist assumptions about human sexuality, the supposed objectivity of their research findings, their empiricism, and the apparent value neutrality of their scientific research. This social constructionist framework, however, is necessarily grounded in explicitly realist philosophical assumptions in order to preserve the possibility of objective knowledge while avoiding the problem of relativism.

The study itself is based on documentary research, analysis and evaluation of both primary and secondary sources. It involved a systematic analysis and evaluation of Masters and Johnson's (1966; 1970) major texts, *Human Sexual Response* and *Human Sexual Inadequacy*. It also involved the study of a number of other works by Masters and Johnson which helped to shed light on aspects of their sex research or sex therapy program (e.g., Masters and Johnson 1976; Masters and Johnson 1979; Masters and Johnson 1980; Masters, Johnson and Kolodny 1985; and Masters, Johnson and Kolodny 1994). Research was also conducted by drawing on other primary sources which were relevant to the study of Masters and Johnson, as well as the secondary literature on their work in the areas of education, feminism, history, medicine, philosophy, psychiatry, psychology, sexology, sex therapy and sociology. A significant proportion of the documentary research in this study took the form of historical research using published sources of information to reconstruct some of the unknown history of the sociology of sex.

The book consists of eight chapters, including this introduction. Chapter 2 is partly concerned with accounting for the nature and dearth of previous sociological attention to Masters and Johnson's (1966; 1970) work. In addressing this issue, it challenges the 'conventional' view of the history of the sociology of sex, and argues for a new interpretation of that history.

Chapter 3 reviews and evaluates two of the major theoretical perspectives on human sexuality: essentialism and social constructionism. While the chapter is critical of aspects of both perspectives, and their application to the study and understanding of human sexuality, it argues for the use of a social constructionist perspective, grounded in realist philosophy, in this book.

Chapter 4 is concerned with Masters and Johnson's (1966) laboratory research on human sexual response. It reviews and analyses the rationale, conduct, major findings and public impact of this research. It argues, in part, that there was a generally favourable response to Masters and Johnson's research and that, when it was criticised, the criticism was more concerned with the methods rather than the findings of their research.

Chapter 5 provides a critique of the centrepiece of Masters and Johnson's (1966) research on sexual physiology: their four stage model of the human sexual response cycle. The chapter criticises their claims about the originality of their model, the strongly essentialist assumptions on which it is based, inconsistencies between their model and their reported data on sexual response, their ideological emphasis on the sexual similarities of males and females, and their inaccurate research findings.

Chapter 6 provides a critique of Masters and Johnson's (1970) concept and classification (or nosology) of sexual dysfunction. It criticises the nosology for its reliance on a model of healthy sexual functioning which has limited generalisability as a set of clinical norms; its gender biases in the classification of sexual dysfunctions; its hetero-coital bias; its inability to deal with possible problems concerning sexual desire; its medicalisation of deviant sexual response; and its tendency to conflate sexual dysfunctions with sexual problems.

Chapter 7 critically discusses the principles, practices and effectiveness of Masters and Johnson's (1970) sex therapy program. It argues, in part, that much of this program was based on the unacknowledged principles and techniques of behaviour therapy, that the effectiveness of their treatment program could not be ascertained from their published study of it, and that the program itself tended to implicitly operate as an institution of social control.

Finally, chapter 8 concludes the book by summing up the main argument, and briefly noting some of the implications for contemporary sex therapy.

2 The Sociology of Sex in Historical Perspective

INTRODUCTION

The research for this chapter developed from an attempt to explain the relative lack of sociological attention to Masters and Johnson's (1966; 1970) work in the forty odd years since they first published *Human Sexual Response*. After reviewing the small sociological literature about them, and reading conventional accounts of the history of the sociology of sex, the explanation as to why sociologists had largely ignored Masters and Johnson initially seemed clear. Sociology, for most of its history, had apparently ignored the study of sexuality altogether, and this naturally included the work of Masters and Johnson. Furthermore, since sociologists claimed that the sociology of sex first developed in the 1960s or early 1970s, (around the same time that Masters and Johnson published *Human Sexual Response* and *Human Sexual Inadequacy*), it could also have been argued that the sociology of sex was too immature to offer any kind of distinctive or critical analysis of their work. If these views were correct then apparently all that remained to be done, in terms of this part of my research, was to document and expound the evidence supporting these propositions.

However, my research on the sociology of sex led me to reject the conventional history of it, and the way it might have accounted for the neglect of Masters and Johnson's work. The conventional view is that there was little or no sociological study of sexuality before World War II, and that a sociology of sex only emerged in the postwar era, and, in some accounts, as late as the 1960s or early 1970s. In the conventional view, there are various 'explanations' for this but it is often 'explained' by referring to the way in which sex research was stifled and inhibited by a repressive society. The apparent emergence of a sociology of sex in the postwar era was also 'explained' in terms of the lifting of repression and the greater opportunities for sociologists to study sexuality.

In this chapter, I criticise the conventional view of the history of the sociology of sex, and argue that sociology was part of the discursive explosion about sexuality that occurred in Western societies from the eighteenth century. Much of this chapter is taken up with documenting the largely unknown history of the sociology of sex from the 1840s to 1960, particularly focusing on sociology in the United States. My aim here is not to write a comprehensive history of the sociology of sex. To my knowledge, no such history has yet been written, and while this is undoubtedly a very important task, it is clearly beyond the scope of this chapter. My aims, in the first part of this chapter, are to provide sufficient evidence that sociology *was* part of the discursive explosion about sexuality that characterised Western societies from the eighteenth century, to sketch some of its main contours, and to discuss some of the reasons why it took the course that it did.

I then discuss the reasons why sociologists have largely misunderstood the history of their discipline's sex research. I argue that the rise of the classical canon in sociology altered many sociologists' conceptions of their discipline, its history, and the kind of topics which were thought to be important for sociological study.

I then examine the nature of the limited sociological literature on Masters and Johnson's (1966; 1970) work and explain why sociologists have largely ignored it. My explanation centres on the rise of the classical canon in sociology, the hegemonic biomedical and clinical definitions of their work, and the perceived quality and importance of their sex research and therapy.

After discussing some of the reasons why most of the main sociological critiques of Masters and Johnson's (1966; 1970) work have occurred from around 1980 and after, I conclude the chapter by highlighting the need for a more comprehensive sociological analysis of their work than previously exists. The chapter begins, however, with an outline of Foucault's (1981) critique of the 'repressive hypothesis' about the history of Western sexuality which has parallels with my own argument.

DOES SOCIOLOGY HAVE ITS OWN VERSION OF THE 'REPRESSIVE HYPOTHESIS'?

In his influential work, *The History of Sexuality* (Volume 1), the French scholar Michel Foucault (1981) attacks what he calls the 'repressive hypothesis' about the history of Western sexuality. According to this hypothesis, the relative sexual freedom allowed to people in their speech and behaviour prior to the seventeenth century in Europe was increasingly repressed from the seventeenth century onward with the development of capitalist society and the later ascendancy of the Victorian bourgeoisie. The extent of this repression was said to be so great, and with so few spaces for escape, that even after nearly three more centuries people were still struggling to liberate their sexuality from this repression. Sexual repression in this account was basically explained by the demands of capitalist society for exploitable labour power. Labour power was said to be sexually regulated so that its energies were not dissipated by the pursuit of pleasure in itself but used only as a means to reproduce more workers (Foucault 1981, Part One).

In arguing against the repressive hypothesis, Foucault does not deny that there were prohibitions, hesitations and prudishness concerning sexual speech and conduct but considers these phenomena as secondary in relation to the enormous expansion in the number of discourses about sexuality from the eighteenth century. He argued that 'Surely no other type of society has ever accumulated — and in such a relatively short span of time — a similar quantity of discourses concerned with sex' (Foucault 1981, 33). These discourses were Foucault's (1981, 69) primary research interest and he wrote that 'the history of sexuality... must first be written from the viewpoint of a history of discourses.'

Many sociological writers on sexuality seem to subscribe to their own version of a repressive hypothesis about the historical relationship between their own discipline and the field of human sexuality. In the first place, there is a common and almost unchallenged view among these sociologists that their discipline has largely ignored the study and analysis of sexuality throughout its history (see, for example, Bowman 1949, 625–6; Reiss 1967, 1–2; Sagarin 1971, 382–4; Plummer 1975, 3; DeLamater 1981, 263; Stein 1989, 5; Tiryakian 1990, 191; Irvine, 1994, 232–3; Seidman 1994b, 166–9; Marshall 1994, 473; Richardson 2001; Gamson and Moon 2004; and Scott and Marshall 2005). This view is well encapsulated by Plummer (1975, 3) who, over thirty years ago, wrote that 'Sociologists have failed to study a most important aspect of human social conduct: that of sexuality....[and] few sociologists have shown any interest in this field.'

A corollary of this view is the belief that when sociologists did begin to study and analyse human sexuality it was relatively late in the discipline's history. The sociologists who espouse these views usually agree that there was little or no sociology of sex before World War II. This is well exemplified in Sagarin's (1971, 384) comment that 'the period from the Darwinian revolution to the Second World War was quite barren of any sociology of sex, [Kingsley] Davis being the most noteworthy exception....' These sociologists, however, disagree about when the sociology of sex first developed or became prominent. Some writers date the emergence of the sociology of sex from the social survey research of Alfred Kinsey and his colleagues published in 1948 and 1953 (Reiss 1967, 2; Sagarin 1971, 385; Ruefli 1985, 189); some date it more vaguely to the 'postwar era' which seems to mean somewhere between the 1950s and the 1970s (Stein 1989, 5; Seidman 1994b, 168-9; Wilton 2000, 66-71; Gamson and Moon 2004); some date it from the 1960s (Marshall 1994, 473; Scott and Marshall 2005), the mid to late 1960s (DeLamater 1981, 263; Richardson 2001), or the early 1970s (Plummer 1983, 351). Others write that sexuality has only been a 'fashionable area of theoretical debate' in sociology since the mid-1970s (Jackson 1993, 201); or publish chapters, in the late 1970s with titles like

'Toward the sociology of sex' as if sociology had yet to study or understand anything about sexuality (Henslin 1978, 1).

Sociologists often try to explain the alleged lack of a sociology of sex before the 'postwar era' by claiming or implying that there was a kind of repression operating within society (or within sociologists themselves) which discouraged or prevented them from studying sexuality. There are variations of this view but, in the main, it can be summarised as follows: the taboo or illegitimate nature of sexuality could create problems for researchers because their social conditioning or moral beliefs might forbid them from studying the topic; their motives could be questioned; they could be subject to 'personal attacks and abuse'; they risked their personal and professional reputations, their jobs and careers; they risked infringing the law; they risked relevant authorities refusing to co-operate with them; they risked funding bodies refusing to finance their research; they risked potential research participants refusing to become involved in the research or refusing to talk about such a sensitive topic; they risked publishers refusing to publish reports of their work; and they risked negative peer review and public censure of their work if it was published (see, for example, Bowman 1949, 625–6; Gebhard 1968, 392; Sagarin 1971, 379–80; Plummer 1975, 4; McKinney 1986, 120; Schneider and Gould 1987, 120–1; and Irvine 1994, 233). In this respect, Plummer (1975, 5) has commented that 'While in other areas of life, the search for understanding through research is seen as the *sine qua non* of progress, in sexual matters it is decried as irrelevant, dehumanizing and pernicious' (emphasis in original).

Apart from explanations which emphasise repression, sociologists have also put forward alternative (though sometimes related) explanations for the lack of a sociology of sex. These include, for example, the explanation that other intellectual traditions or disciplines, such as biomedicine, psychoanalysis and the social survey tradition out-competed sociology for 'ownership' of sexuality and thereby came to dominate the field (Reiss 1967, 1, 3; Sagarin 1971, 382, 384; Plummer 1975, 3; Marshall 1994, 473); that the dominance of the biomedical and psychoanalytic traditions created or reinforced the belief that sexuality was a natural, biological, psychological and/or individual phenomenon unsuited to sociological study (Sagarin 1971, 384; Plummer 1975, 5; Vance 1989, 13–15; Epstein 1994, 189–190; Seidman 1994b, 167); that sociologists had more difficulty justifying their research on sexuality than other groups with similar interests, such as doctors, psychologists, anthropologists and journalists (Reiss 1967, 2–3); and that sex research had low status in the academic hierarchy and was devalued by sociologists, funding bodies, publishers and the wider society (Plummer 1975, 4).

Although many sociologists have tried to explain the lack of a sociology of sex, few have tried to explain why a sociology of sex allegedly developed during the 'postwar era.' When they did try to explain it, their explanations consisted of three main points. Firstly, a sociology of sex developed because the fetters on sociological sex research had been broken by the impact of the earlier sex research of Kinsey, and Masters and Johnson, and by the growing liberalisation of public attitudes to sexuality. Secondly, sociology was able to take advantage of this greater freedom because the discipline had become more mature in its development. Thirdly, sociologists' interest in studying and writing about sex was stimulated by social changes which led to the loosening of sexual mores in the 1950s, and sexual rebellion in the 1960s (see, for example, the explanations put forward by Reiss 1967, 3–4; Sagarin 1971, 393, 395–7; and Seidman 1994b, 167–9).

BEYOND THE REPRESSIVE HYPOTHESIS: SOCIOLOGY AND THE DISCURSIVE EXPLOSION ABOUT SEXUALITY

Like Foucault (1981), one of my aims in this chapter is not to deny that there was repression in the past which discouraged or prevented sociologists or other researchers from conducting or publishing sex research. Indeed, there appear to be many instances where this happened (see, for example, Burgess 1939a; Ehrmann 1964, 607–8; Suggs and Marshall 1971, 220–1; Martinson 1973, vii; LoPiccolo and Heiman 1977; Pomeroy 1982; Bullough 1985; Davis and Whitten 1987, 69, 72; Troiden 1987; Kon 1993, Ch. 1; Bullough 1994a, 74–5; Okami and Pendleton 1994, 85–6; Irvine 2005, Afterword). Even as late as the 1980s and 1990s, political interference in national sex research surveys in Britain and the United States led to a withdrawal of government funding for these projects. Both were subsequently completed with funding from private foundations (Johnson, Wadsworth, Wellings and Field 1994; Laumann, Gagnon, Michael and Michaels 1994; Laumann, Michael and Gagnon 1994; Michaels and Giami 1999, 401). Nor do I deny that there may be periods in a society's history where there is greater or lesser sexual repression which may have an effect, among other things, on the opportunities to conduct and publish sex research (see, for example, Brecher 1970; Gagnon 1975; Robinson 1976; LoPiccolo and Heiman 1977; Kon 1993, Ch.1; Bullough 1994a, 74–5).

Rather, one of my aims in this chapter is to argue for a different way of looking at sociology's relationship with sexuality. Instead of seeing sociology as largely ignoring the study of sexuality for most of its history, I want to argue, in a manner similar to Foucault (1981) and Sydie (1994, 117), that sociology was part of the discursive explosion about sexuality that characterised Western societies from the eighteenth century.

Early figures associated with the development of sociology, such as Karl Marx and Friedrich Engels, Auguste Comte and Herbert Spencer, all addressed themselves, at least in part, and in varying ways to topics of a sexual nature. Karl Marx (1818–1883), the German critic of political economy, did not identify himself as a sociologist but much of his work was later incorporated (not always accurately) into sociology, and he is now generally regarded as a 'founder' of the discipline. He and Friedrich Engels, his friend and collaborator, are not usually known for their writings about human sexuality. (A possible exception may be Engels's 1902 [1884] *The Origin of the Family, Private Property and the State).* Yet, they made many interesting observations and comments about it. For example, Marx wrote about how sex as a natural species power could become socialised or humanised. Furthermore, he thought the extent of this socialisation or humanisation was an important indicator of human self-development. He and Engels also wrote about the alienated sexuality of bourgeois marriage and prostitution, sexuality under communism, and the need to understand historically the social relations of human sexual reproduction (Marx 1956 [1932]; Marx and Engels 1947 [1932]; Marx and Engels 1956 [1845]; Marx and Engels 1967 [1848]; Kern 1975, ch.6; Ollman 1971; Ollman 1977).

Auguste Comte (1798–1857), the man who famously coined the term 'sociology', also wrote about sex in his *System of Positive Polity*, first published between 1851 and 1854. He believed the sexual instinct could be 'satisfied and disciplined' in marriage leading to marital harmony while sexual freedom would result in social disorder. He thought the main purpose of marriage was to morally educate people toward universal love defined as the 'subjection of self-interest to social feeling...' (Comte 1975 [1851–1854], 377). He explained that if the goal of moral education was to be achieved then marriage had to be monogamous and permanent. This was because 'Love cannot be deep unless it remains constant to a fixed object, for the very possibility of change is a temptation to it' (Comte 1975 [1851-1854], 377). He then explained the connection between personal and universal love: 'From personal experience of strong love we rise by degrees to sincere affection for all mankind strong enough to modify conduct, although, as the scope widens, its energy must decrease' (Comte 1975 [1851–1854], 377). Comte (1975 [1851–1854], 377) held that the moral education of marriage (and the disciplining of sexual love) could provide a basis for individual and public welfare, and that the superiority of social life in Western societies was probably due more to monogamy than to any other cause.

Finally, the British sociologist, Herbert Spencer (1820–1903), analysed 'the passion that unites the sexes' (Spencer 1970 [1855], 601). He considered this passion to be 'the most compound, and therefore the most powerful, of all the feelings' (Spencer 1970 [1855], 601). He analysed it into nine different elements: the physical elements of sexual attraction; impressions of beauty; feelings of affection; sentiments of admiration and respect; feelings of being preferred and admired 'above all the world' 'by one admired beyond all others'; feelings of self-esteem, boosted by gaining a desirable partner and having sway over him or her; proprietary feelings or the pleasure of possessing such a desirable partner; the love of unrestrained activity with a partner in the absence of personal barriers; and the doubling of personal pleasures by sharing them with an intimate other. Spencer (1970

[1855] 601–2) believed the physical feelings were the 'nucleus of the whole' but that the mutual excitement of the various related emotions fused them into an immense aggregation of passion with 'irresistible power'.

IMPERIALISM AND THE INSTITUTIONALISATION OF SOCIOLOGY IN THE UNIVERSITIES

Early 'sociological' figures, such as Marx and Engels, Comte, and Spencer, were often writing about sex in the mid-nineteenth century or earlier. Sociology had not yet become institutionalised as a teaching discipline in the universities. This generally occurred in the period from 1880–1910 in the large cities and university towns of France, Germany, Britain, the United States and Russia (Connell 1997, 1515). This was the period when the first chairs of sociology were created and professors appointed, the first named sociology departments and undergraduate courses established, and sociological associations and journals founded. By the beginning of World War I, these institutions were established in most European countries and the United States (Connell 1997, 1528).

This was also a period of major European and United States' imperial expansion which Connell (1997, 1511) argues 'gave sociology its main conceptual framework, and much of its data, key problems and methods.' He argues, for example, that imperialism facilitated the flow of information back from the colonies and allowed European and North American sociologists to compare and contrast, from the outside, a vast range of different societies. As well as the sweeping use of the comparative method, sociologists also relied on 'grand ethnography' for holistic accounts of entire societies (Connell 1997, 1525–6).

The existence of major differences between societies had to be explained and the theoretical framework which 'dominated all debates from the 1860s to the 1920s was an evolutionary one' (Weeks 1985, 99). Sociologists sought to understand, firstly, the difference between their own 'civilised' societies and the 'primitiveness' of other societies; and, secondly, how 'primitive' societies progressed to become more 'advanced'. In order to explain this apparent process of evolution, sociologists borrowed ideas from 'Victorian biological and social thought' (Connell 1997, 1517). The main debate centred on whether the contrast between the primitive and the civilised should be explained in terms of 'physical evolution from lower to higher human types or through an evolution of mind and social forms and whether competition or cooperation was the motor of progress' (Suggs and Miracle 1993, 483; Connell 1997, 1520). One reason for the use of 'grand ethnography' was to provide holistic accounts of those societies believed to be 'at the origin and the end of progress' (Connell 1997, 1525–6). This was done on the assumption that archaic society was fundamentally different to modern society. Tonnies's (1955 [1887]) famous contrast between *gemeinschaft* ('community') and *gesellschaft* ('society or association') was but one example of this.

Connell (1997, 1521) argues that the substantive topics addressed by sociologists at this time were also bound up with issues of empire and colonisation. Although early sociological attention to issues of class, alienation and industrialisation is often emphasised in conventional histories of the discipline, 'race', gender and sexuality were all core issues in early sociology. The social relations of empire required attention to the topic of 'race' and the concern of sociologists 'with evolutionary progress and hierarchies of populations' similarly required attention to issues of gender and sexuality (Connell 1997, 1521).

In the period from 1880 to the early 1920s, many sociologists in Europe and the United States wrote about sexuality. Their treatment of the topic was often affected by imperialism and evolutionary thinking although in some cases it was influenced more by developments in their own countries (Connell 1997, 1522).

In France, Charles Letourneau and Emile Durkheim both examined the topic. Letourneau (1881) drew on studies of animal sexuality and ethnographic material from around the world to describe, rank and 'explain' 'racial' and gender differences in relation to such matters as the strength and expression of the genesic (sexual) instinct, sexual licentiousness, prostitution, adultery and sodomy. He argued that 'from the age of primitive barbarism' there had been a gradual evolution of human moral refinement in relation to sexual matters and that the white races were 'incontestably more advanced than other races both in intelligence and in morality...' (Letourneau 1881, 69, 73). Durkheim tackled sexuality in a range of works including a book on suicide, a lengthy article on the nature and origins of the incest taboo, a short review of a work on primitive marriage, an argument against a proposal for divorce by mutual consent, a discussion of sex education, and a book on *The Elementary Forms of the Religious Life* (Durkheim 1963 [1897]; Durkheim 1970 [1897]; Durkheim 1976 [1912]; Durkheim 1979 [1911]; Tiryakian 1990).

The Finnish sociologist and philosopher Edward Westermarck (1891) also examined many aspects of human sexuality in his reputation-making *The History of Human Marriage*. His discussion of sexuality was central to his thesis that monogamy was the original form of human marriage and that early human beings did not live in a state of sexual promiscuity.

In Germany, sociologists such as Ferdinand Tonnies, Georg Simmel and Max Weber all addressed themselves to topics of a sexual nature. In *Gemeinschaft and Gesellschaft*, Tonnies (1955 [1887], 5, 43, 55) discussed some of the reasons for love at first sight, the ways that sexual relationships between men and women needed to be strengthened to stop the sexual subordination of women (who he regarded as naturally weaker than men), and the way that loving marital relationships formed a cornerstone of gemeinschaft. Georg Simmel regularly wrote 'on issues concerning women, sexuality and love' throughout his career (Oakes 1984a, vii). As early as 1892, in a treatise on ethical theory, Simmel wrote about the relationship between women, money and prostitution, a topic he returned to in *The Philosophy of Money* in 1900. He also wrote essays on flirtation and love, and dealt with male and female sexuality in an essay entitled 'The relative and absolute in the problem of the sexes' (Oakes 1984a; Oakes 1984b; Simmel 1984). Similarly, Max Weber (1970), in a number of different works between 1915 and 1921, discussed sex and marriage among the Hindu castes, including the Kulin Brahmans; the sexual prerogatives of the members of bachelor houses under warrior communism; religious orgies; and the way in which processes of 'rationalisation' could transform sexual love, 'the greatest irrational force in life,' into routinised sexual desires and practices (Weber 1970, 343).

In the United States, sexuality was addressed both by 'social evolutionist' sociologists, such as Lester Ward and William Graham Sumner, and by first generation members of the 'Chicago School' of sociology, such as W. I. Thomas, Charles Henderson and Graham Taylor. Ward was the first president of the American Sociological Society and Sumner taught the first course that could be called sociology in the United States. Both were influenced, although in different degrees, by Herbert Spencer's 'Social Darwinist' ideas (Ritzer 1996, 45–6). Ward (1903) developed a sociology of sex and gender in his book *Pure Sociology* and spent 127 pages discussing the influence exerted by the phylogenetic forces: 'forces that have reproduction for their functional end in the direction of creating and transforming social structures' (Ward 1903, 290). In the course of this discussion, Ward examined a range of topics from sex and reproduction, to gender relations, marriage and different types of love. Sumner's (1959 [1906], 2) last and most influential major work, *Folkways,* was an attempt to give an overview of 'all that we have learned from anthropology and ethnography about primitive men and primitive society.' Much of the book was concerned with gender relations and sexual customs with chapters on sex mores, marriage, incest and sacral harlotry.

Early members of the Chicago School were also writing about sexuality in the period between 1907 and World War I. W. I. Thomas's (1907) book *Sex and Society* was primarily concerned with sex and gender but still touched on topics such as sexual interest, courtship, sexual activity, reproduction and sexual perversion. Charles Henderson headed the Chicago Society for Social Hygiene which worked to control venereal disease and promote sex education. He published a handbook in 1909 called *Education With Reference to Sex* which was a major resource for the early sex education movement. The main aim of this movement was to endorse the repression of all non-procreative sexual activity (Sprague 1990, 70, 72). Finally, Graham Taylor, a member of the Chicago Vice Commission provided social science research for the Commission by interviewing prostitutes and visiting brothels. The Commission's 400-page report *The Social*

Evil in Chicago (1911) aimed to abolish commercial prostitution and recommend that governments introduce 'tougher laws to suppress all forms of illicit sexuality' (Sprague 1990, 76). Taylor also delivered a paper on the 'Public repression of social evil' to the First National Conference on Race Betterment in 1914. Here, he argued, in part, that the strong sexual passions of men and low wages for women led to the development of female prostitution. Taylor believed the government should take responsibility for controlling men's unruly sexual passions if men could not or would not control them themselves (Sprague 1990, 71, 79).

THE IMPACT OF WORLD WAR I

World War I fractured the relationships between the sociological communities which had been developing in Europe and the United States. A number of key sociologists on different sides of the conflict broke off contact with their foreign colleagues and devoted themselves to their countries' respective war efforts. At the same time, the brutality and carnage of the war undermined the previously taken for granted notion that social evolution involved a progressive increase in civilisation and rational conduct. 'The foundation of sociology's worldview was ruptured' (Connell 1997, 1533). Institutional stagnation followed with sociological groups losing their way and dispersing or vainly trying to resurrect the social evolutionist program. In the decade around 1920, this program irretrievably broke down (Connell 1997, 1534).

New forms of sociology which could have replaced the evolutionary approach were stifled in Europe by the 'balance of global power and the growth of totalitarianism' (Connell 1997, 1535). However, an alternative form of academic sociology emerged in the United States between 1920 and 1950. Compared to the older evolutionist sociology, it 'had a different object of knowledge, a new set of methods and applications, a revised definition of the discipline, a new audience, and — eventually — a new view of its history' (Connell 1997, 1535).

Its new object of knowledge was society (particularly the sociologists' own societies) and, more specifically, social problems and social disorder within these societies. These issues had been studied to some extent by earlier sociologists but they had been 'intellectually subordinated...to... conceptions of global difference and evolutionary progress' (Connell 1997, 1535). They now 'became the intellectual center of sociology' (Connell 1997, 1535).

New statistical techniques for analysing quantitative data were developed and applied primarily to survey data and the collection of official statistics, particularly in the United States. A new empiricist zeal guided and underpinned the collection and assemblage of facts. In the 1920s and 1930s, empirical research accelerated on the social life of America's suburbs, towns and cities, underpinned by large increases in government and corporate funding of sociological research. At the same time, sociologists' conceptions of their discipline generally changed from the Comtean vision of sociology as a metascience to sociology as one social science among others. In defining what sociology's new and special focus was 'no formulation was very convincing, and none became generally accepted' (Connell 1997, 1537).

THE SOCIOLOGY OF SEX IN THE INTER-WAR YEARS

During the inter-war years, the social survey or 'book-keeping' tradition became a more prominent part of sociological sex research. It was primarily concerned with understanding and solving sociosexual 'problems' rather than with developing or testing social theory. It largely addressed itself to understanding two major 'problems' concerning heterosexuality: the increasing premarital sexual activity of young people and the problems of couples with sexual adjustment in marriage (Ehrmann 1963, 145; Ehrmann 1964, 598). The survey researchers came from a range of disciplines and occupations, including sociology, biology, psychology, psychiatry and journalism, but they collected important data on the social determinants of sexual behaviour. They usually collected their data from self-selected respondents by means of questionnaires or interviews, and the data were then statistically analysed and interpreted (Ehrmann 1963, 143; Ehrmann 1964, 598; Gagnon 1975, 122–3).

The first known surveys of sexual practices in the United States began in the 1890s. They were conducted by Clelia Mosher (a biology student and later a physician) and Robert Latou Dickinson (an obstetrician-gynaecologist) who collected their data by means of questionnaires. However, most of Dickinson's 'statistical data was not published until the early 1930s, and Mosher's study was not published until 1974 (Degler 1984; Bullough 1994b, 308–11). Kinsey et al (1948, 24) credit Exner's (1915) study of the sex education and behaviour of 948 male college students as 'the pioneer attempt to secure statistical data on American sexual behavior' but probably because of World War I, no similar major studies on sex were published for almost fifteen years (Ehrmann 1964, 598).

Research on love and marriage (including sex), however, became more feasible after the war. Burgess and Wallin (1953, 34) argue that the principal reason for this was a change in attitudes to the increasing divorce rate. Experts and the public no longer believed that the 'problem' of divorce could be solved by making divorce more difficult to legally obtain. They realised that there were many factors both before and after marriage which contributed to its success or failure. Psychologists and sociologists became interested in the question of whether they could predict success or failure in marriage and focused their research on the 'adjustment of two persons in interaction with each other in courtship and marriage' (Burgess and Wallin 1953, 34). Following Exner's (1915) research, other significant studies in this tradition, prior to World War II, included Davis's (1929) *Factors in the Sex Life of Twenty-Two Hundred Women*, Hamilton's (1986 [1929]) *A Research in Marriage*, Dickinson and Beam's (1970 [1931]) *A Thousand Marriages*, Terman and colleagues' (1938) *Psychological Factors in Marital Happiness*, Bromley and Britten's (1938) *Youth and Sex*, and Landis and colleagues' (1940) *Sex in Development*. According to Gagnon (1975, 123), these kinds of early studies produced at least a partial picture of middle class sexual behaviour. They showed:

> conventional individuals trying to work out their own sexual lives in a situation of profound personal ignorance, misinformation, and cultural isolation.... The picture of sex in marriage that emerged from this early research was a history of fumbling and often mute struggles to find some sense of order, an attempt to place sexuality in some reasonable relationship to the rest of life and make sense of the changing relations between the genders. (Gagnon 1975, 123)

Gagnon (1975, 121–2) argues that these early studies of sexual behaviour did not have a 'deep collective influence' on social scientists, academics and sexual reformers. However, they were important because they anticipated changes to the style and content of sex research. Firstly, they anticipated the use of scientific sampling, standardised questionnaires and the presentation of data in statistical and tabular form. This foreshadowed later survey research on sexual behaviour, such as the Kinsey reports (1948 and 1953), and contrasted with much of the earlier sex research which relied on case histories. Secondly, they involved relatively 'normal' or 'conventional' population samples rather than the 'exotic and the curious, the neurotic, or the criminal' (Gagnon 1975, 121).

As sociology transformed itself as a discipline, members of the Chicago School continued their studies of urban social 'problems,' including those directly and indirectly concerned with human sexuality. First generation members of the School, such as W. I. Thomas and Graham Taylor both published work in the 1920s and 1930s. Thomas (1969 [1923]), for example, produced a sociological study of delinquency — *The Unadjusted Girl* — in which he wrote about the causes, social context and nature of female prostitution. Taylor published *Pioneering On Social Frontiers* in 1930 in which he argued that the lack of sex education made urban young people vulnerable to the social forces promoting illicit sexuality (Sprague 1990, 71).

The second generation of Chicago School sociologists, and their postgraduate students, continued to work on topics such as urban social problems and sexuality. Ernest Burgess (1926; 1939a; 1939b), for example, published articles on 'The romantic impulse and family disorganization'

(1926), 'The influence of Sigmund Freud upon sociology in the United States' (1939b) and 'Three pioneers in the study of sex' (1939a). He also wrote a book with Leonard Cottrell, Jr. — *Predicting Success or Failure in Marriage* — in which they looked at marital adjustment as a social problem and examined the role of changing sex mores on such adjustments (Burgess and Cottrell, Jr. 1939). In the 1920s and 1930s, Burgess's and Robert Park's graduate students were also involved in studying 'illicit' sexual behaviour. Harvey Zorbaugh (1929), for example, in his book, *The Gold Coast and the Slum*, wrote about free love, promiscuity, unmarried men and women living together, homosexuality and prostitution within the urban area he studied. Similarly, Paul Cressey (1969 [1932]), in his study of the taxi-dance hall, wrote about the sexual philosophy and practices of the female taxi-dancers, their 'sex games' with men, their forms of sexual alliance, their romantic impulses and promiscuity, and the relationship between the taxi-dance hall and prostitution. Sprague (1990, 77) notes that many of these studies contained a 'restrained moral condemnation' of the sexual behaviour they studied and implied that such behaviour was pathological. He argues that, in effect, they 'continued to support the old moral code of Protestant America' (Sprague 1990, 77).

Another scholar at the University of Chicago who emphasised the importance of sex for understanding society was George Herbert Mead. Mead was a social psychologist who became one of the founders of symbolic interactionist sociology. In one of his most famous books, *Mind, Self and Society*, published posthumously in 1934, Mead (1962 [1934], 227–8) wrote that basic biological impulses such as for food and sex, are broadly:

> social in character or have social implications, since they involve or require social situations and relations for their satisfaction by any given individual organism; and they constitute the foundation of all types... of social behavior, however simple or complex, crude or highly organized....

He held that the 'sex or reproductive impulse' was the most important of the 'fundamental socio-physiological impulses' for human social behaviour and that it 'most decisively or determinately expresses itself in the whole general form of human social organization...' (Mead 1962 [1934], 228).

A final example of sociological sex research in the 1930s can be provided with the work of Edward Westermarck. He published four books — *Ethical Relativity* (1970 [1932]), *Three Essays on Sex and Marriage* (1934), *The Future of Marriage in Western Civilization* (1936), and *Christianity and Morals* (1939) — which dealt with human sexuality to a greater or lesser degree, and covered such specific topics as Freud's views on the oedipus complex, sexual maladjustment in marriage, adultery, and 'Christianity and irregular sex relations' (Westermarck 1934; 1936; 1939; 1970 [1932]).

THE FAILURE OF EMPIRICISM AND THE RE-MAKING OF SOCIOLOGY IN TERMS OF THE 'CLASSICAL CANON'

By the 1930s, it was clear that the main strands of empiricism in U.S. sociology had reached an intellectual and disciplinary impasse. They had failed to provide a fruitful and expanding research program for the discipline and failed to win a significant proportion of U.S. sociologists to their cause. The American Sociological Society was split by bitter empiricist, and other in-fighting, and funding began to dry up (Bannister 1987, 7, 190, 237; Connell 1997, 1537). At this point, there was an attempt by some sociologists to reconstruct their discipline. The reconstruction centred on the creation of a 'canon': a set of privileged texts exemplifying 'classical sociology' whose interpretation and reinterpretation would define the discipline (Connell 1997, 1512, 1545).

Connell (1997, 1537) argues that this process of canon making had three main elements. Firstly, it involved the construction of a canonical point of view: sociology was newly conceived as being founded by a small group of brilliant intellectuals who were trying to understand social changes internal to European and North American societies caused by the development of capitalism, and the Industrial and French revolutions. Yet Connell (1997, 1516) argues that most sociological research, treatises, and textbooks, before World War I, were not primarily concerned with the social structures of European and North American societies or their modernisation. Rather, sociology 'was formed within the culture of imperialism' and this strongly affected both its research methods and content (Connell 1997, 1519).

Secondly, the process of canon making involved the selection of particular intellectuals (and not others) as belonging to the elite group of sociology's founders. There was not always agreement on which sociologists were the founders, and there were a variety of factors involved in the choice and elevation of particular figures. Many contemporary and recent sociological textbooks list Karl Marx, Max Weber and Emile Durkheim as the main founders of sociology with other figures, such as Auguste Comte, Herbert Spencer and Georg Simmel playing a secondary role. Yet Connell (1997, 1514) argues that, before World War II, most sociologists saw the development of their discipline as a collective enterprise involving the labour of many different scholars — including those now in the modern canon — in the advancement of scientific knowledge. There was also little sense that certain classic texts defined sociology and deserved special study. 'It was only in the following generation that the idea of a classical period and the short list of classical authors and canonical texts took hold' (Connell 1997, 1514).

Thirdly, the process of canon making involved the dissemination of the 'founders'' writings and ideas to students and practitioners of sociology. This process was facilitated, from the 1930s, by the systematic translation of key European sociological texts into English. These texts included

Weber's (1985 [1904–1905]) *The Protestant Ethic and the Spirit of Capitalism*, and Durkheim's (1964 [1894]) *The Rules of Sociological Method*. These translations provided source material for sociologists to develop the teaching of 'classical sociology' in U.S. graduate education after World War II (Connell 1997, 1543).

The process of canon making would last a generation and involve the labour of many different sociologists, including such notables as Talcott Parsons, Robert Merton and C. Wright Mills. However, as Connell (1997) argues, and as we shall see later, the fulfilment of this project by the early 1960s would have profound consequences for sociology's understanding of itself and its own history. In particular, it would have important consequences for sociology's understanding of its past in relation to research and writing about sexuality.

SOCIOLOGICAL SEX RESEARCH AND WORLD WAR II

World Wat II began in 1939 and was to last for almost six years. During this time, in the United States, social survey research on sexuality virtually stopped but other sociological research on sexuality continued (Ehrmann, 1964, 598). Examples of journal articles on sexuality published during this time include Ellis's (1939) 'Freud's influence on the changed attitude toward sex,' Riemer's (1940) 'A research note on incest', Hulett Jr.'s (1940) 'Social role and personal security in Mormon polygamy,' Whyte's (1943) 'A slum sex code,' Opler's (1943) 'Woman's social status and the forms of marriage,' and Kirkpatrick and Caplow's (1945) 'Courtship in a group of Minnesota students.' Perhaps not surprisingly, some of the articles on sexuality published during or shortly after the war themselves focused on how the war was affecting people's sexual attitudes and behaviour. Examples include Burgess's (1942) 'The effect of war on the American family,' Reckless's (1942) 'The impact of war on crime, delinquency and prostitution,' Bromberg's (1943) 'The effects of the war on crime,' and Elkin's (1946) 'Aggressive and erotic tendencies in army life.'

POSTWAR SOCIOLOGY OF SEX

In the postwar period, in the United States, two main sociological traditions were initially prominent in the study of human sexuality: the social survey tradition and the functionalist tradition which partly drew on psychoanalysis. In the social survey tradition, the most important early postwar studies, which tried to get a representative picture of sexual behaviour in the United States, were by Alfred Kinsey and his colleagues. These studies were published as *Sexual Behavior in the Human Male* in 1948 and *Sexual Behavior in the Human Female* in 1953.

Kinsey was trained in zoology and did not have any sociologists on his staff. However, he consulted with sociologists, among others, during his research, and his work was generally regarded as sociological in its approach to sex (Kinsey et al 1948, 8; Kinsey et al 1953, x; Reiss 1967, 2–3; Sagarin 1971, 385; Plummer 1975, 3; DeLora et al 1977, 11–12; Rue-fli 1985, 189). Kinsey et al (1953, 3) set out on a 'fact-finding survey...to discover what people do sexually, what factors account for their patterns of sexual behavior, how their sexual experiences have affected their lives, and what social significance there may be in each type of behavior'.

Like many previous studies in the survey tradition, Kinsey and his colleagues enquired into premarital and marital heterosexual behaviour. However, they also went on to study other forms of sexual behaviour, such as masturbation, homosexuality and human sexual contacts with animals. These had received only limited attention in earlier studies (Ehrmann 1963, 145). The surveys of 5,300 white American males and 5,940 white American females of different ages, religious denominations, educational levels and geographical locations provided, through structured interviews, most of the statistical data analysed and presented in the two Kinsey reports. Kinsey's sample, however, was not representative of the U.S. population and could not provide a reliable basis for generalising his statistical findings to the wider population (Johnson et al 1994, 3).

The Kinsey team's data nevertheless revealed an incredible diversity of sexual behaviour within their sample which diverged markedly from the dominant social norms of heterosexual procreative intercourse within the context of marriage. Their 'findings served to relativize sexual behavior and debunk notions of pathology, calling into question rigid social norms and laying the foundations for more liberal sex research' (Stein 1989, 6). Their most startling data (for that time) concerned female sexuality, male homosexuality and masturbation. Kinsey and his colleagues' research showed, for example, that women were not just interested in sex for reproductive purposes, and that they could sexually respond and reach orgasm as capably as men. In terms of homosexuality, Kinsey and his colleagues' work challenged the idea that homosexuality and heterosexuality were mutually exclusive sexual categories by showing that one third of men and 13% of women reported reaching orgasm at least once with a partner of the same sex by the age of forty-five. Kinsey's team believed it was better to think of sexual behaviour as existing on a continuum with exclusively homosexual and heterosexual behaviour represented at each end. Finally, the Kinsey team's data challenged 'traditional views about the rarity and danger of masturbation among normal adults, since more than 90% of males and 62% of females reported having masturbated' (Reinisch and Harter 1994, 335; Kinsey et al 1948; Kinsey et al 1953).

The Kinsey team's research report created an uproar when it was first published. Powerful political and religious opposition to the research led to the loss of most of their funding between 1954 and 1956. Under the pressures of trying to find new research funding, a punishing work schedule, and defending his work from attack, Kinsey died in 1956 (Gebhard 1976, 13–17). The Kinsey reports, however, remain an important and enduring part of his legacy. They provided the first broadly based systematic research on American sexual behaviour. '[M]ore than 40 years since the first Kinsey report was published, Kinsey's studies are still the most widely known and cited works on human sexual behavior' (Reinisch and Harter 1994, 334).

The Kinsey team's publication of their first volume on male sexual behaviour in 1948 also stimulated sex research in Britain. In 1949, an independent research organisation called 'Mass-Observation' carried out 'Britain's first national random sample survey of sexual attitudes and behaviour' (Stanley 1996, 97). This was some forty-five years before publication of the supposedly pioneering national random sample survey known as the 'British National Survey of Sexual Attitudes and Lifestyles' (Johnson et al 1994). The Mass-Observation research was known as 'Little Kinsey' within the organisation and funded by the *Sunday Pictorial* newspaper (Stanley 1995, 4; Stanley 2001, 102). Some of the research findings were published contemporaneously in that paper but a completed final book manuscript based on the research was not published at the time. It was only published for the first time in 1995 (Stanley 1995). The final version of the manuscript covered a range of different topics. Chapters of the text were concerned with the facts of life, sex education, birth control, marriage, divorce, sex outside marriage, prostitution, the psychology of sex, sexual morality, and opinion formation. There were also appendices on the sexual attitudes and habits of Mass-Observation's National Panel of Voluntary Observers and on homosexuality (Stanley 1995). Stanley (1995, 6) points out that in 'spite of being a British "first" in the field of sex surveys and receiving a good deal of newspaper and radio publicity at the time it was carried out, "Little Kinsey" is now largely unknown even among specialist researchers'.

In the United States, many other postwar surveys of sexual behaviour were conducted between the first Kinsey Report (1948) and the 1960s, the decade when many sociologists have alleged the sociology of sex was born. These surveys, which collected systematic data on the social determinants of sexual behaviour, included those by Landis, Poffenberger and Poffenberger (1950); Locke (1968 [1951]); Burgess and Wallin (1953); Kanin (1957); Kirkpatrick and Kanin (1957); Kanin and Howard (1958); and Ehrmann (1959). Most of these surveys did little to improve on the flawed methodology of Kinsey et al's (1948; 1953) research (Johnson et al 1994, 3). Modern survey methods were not applied with any frequency to the study of human sexual behaviour until the 1960s and 1970s. Indeed, the first study of sexual attitudes and behaviour in the United States to use a probability sample, representative of the U.S. population, was not until 1967 (Reiss 1967). And even when modern survey methods were used in sexual behaviour research, the studies 'were often small or limited to specific subsets of the population' (Johnson et al 1994, 4).

However, despite the methodological problems with much of this literature, sociologists have often regarded the findings as valuable in the absence of more reliable data. Survey research has allowed sociologists to estimate the frequencies of certain sexual behaviours, to examine correlations between those behaviours and various socio-demographic variables, such as age and sex, and to analyse apparent changes in sexual behaviour over time (Schneider and Gould 1987, 127; Marshall 1994, 473).

The other main sociological tradition concerned with the study of sex, that emerged in the postwar United States, was functionalism. Its views of sexuality, however, were often influenced by psychoanalysis (Stein 1989, 5; Scanzoni and Marsiglio 1992, 1754). Psychoanalysis was originally developed by Sigmund Freud from the end of the nineteenth century and is a psychological perspective and method for understanding and treating psychological disorders (Marshall 1994, 427). Freud's psychoanalytic work helped to legitimise the study of sexuality and popularise the idea of 'the importance of sex in human development' (Bullough 1994c, 222; Sagarin 1971, 381).

Freud used two different conceptions of sexuality in his work (Klein 1976). The first emphasised the role of psychological factors and was concerned with the meanings and values which individuals attached to their erotic experiences. The second construed sexuality as a form of natural biological energy which demanded release. Freud himself did not always clearly distinguish between these two conceptions in his work and it is the latter conception which today is almost always regarded as Freud's view of sexuality. This is also the conception which has most often been incorporated into sociology (Stein 1989, 3).

Freud (1977c [1912]) called this natural biological force the libido and believed that while the libido can be repressed in order to meet social requirements its basic source of energy remains. His theory of human personality centred on the 'fate of the libido' (Bullough 1994c, 222). Freud (1977a [1905]; 1977b [1908]; 1977d [1931]) held that the libido is present soon after birth rather than suddenly emerging at puberty, and that the libido is channelled into particular areas of the body which become eroticised. He argued that individuals pass through certain stages of psychosexual development which he called oral, anal, phallic, latency, puberty and genital. At each stage, he stressed that various conflicts are encountered, and that a person's psychological well-being and future sexual orientation depends on how well these conflicts are resolved. If they are not resolved then he believed that 'fixation' would occur: that is, some libido would remain attached to a particular stage and this would affect adult behaviour. Ideally, in Freud's view, individuals should progress from the immature pleasures associated with the mouth, anus and genitals to the mature pleasures of heterosexual intercourse (Bullough 1994c, 222; O'Connell Davidson and Layder 1994, 11).

Freud's psychoanalytic theories and ideas about sex jarred with more conventional views and often provoked derision and outrage. However, psychoanalysis survived this unfriendly reception. It was officially introduced to the United States in 1909 when Freud and Carl Jung visited Clark University. It went on to become one of the most influential movements in the United States in the twentieth century. Much of the literature on sex in the United States between 1930 and 1960 was dominated by psychoanalytic views and at times no other explanations seemed acceptable (Burgess 1939b; Bullough 1994c, 222–3).

There was also an important strand of the psychoanalytic tradition, the 'Freudian Left,' which had a strong sociological interest in the repression of sexual drives by social institutions, as well as the question of sexual liberation (Robinson 1969). This was represented above all in the work of people like Wilhelm Reich and Herbert Marcuse whose ideas were embraced by the 'new left' in the 'sexual revolution' of the 1960s (McLaren 1999, 180). Giddens (1992, 169, 181) points out that few people today read Reich or Marcuse yet, despite their limitations, they present important visions of a non-repressive social order.

It was not until 1920 and after, however, that psychoanalysis had much influence on American sociology. When it did, that influence was evident in attempts by sociologists to integrate psychoanalytic theory, concepts, methods and findings with those of sociology (Burgess 1939b). This influence extended to functionalism which was a major strand in U.S. postwar sociology. According to Davis (1959, 758–9; emphasis in original), functionalism does 'what *any* science does,' namely it relates one part of a whole system to another and relates the parts to the whole. It does this by 'seeing one part as "performing a function for" or "meeting a need requirement of" the whole... or some part of it' (Davis 1959, 758). In his view, sociology is distinctive from other sciences not because of its method (which it shares with other sciences), but because of its subject 'for it deals with human societies whereas other disciplines deal with other kinds of systems' (Davis 1959, 759).

Functionalism had its sociological roots in the work of Auguste Comte, Herbert Spencer and Emile Durkheim (Ritzer 1992, 94; Swingewood 2000, 137). However, it only emerged as a separate, distinctively labelled, school of thought in sociology and social anthropology during the twentieth century (Baert 1998, 38). It developed in sociology in a context of inter and intradisciplinary struggle. Sociology was trying to re-establish itself as a distinctive and legitimate discipline after the collapse of the evolutionist program around 1920 and the empiricist program in the 1930s (Davis 1959; Bannister 1987; Connell 1997). According to Davis (1959, 768), 'the key fact [in the rise of functionalism] was the absence of a sociological [read functionalist] point of view, and the key problem ...was how to develop and establish this point of view.' Davis (1959) identified the main obstacles to establishing a functionalist perspective in sociology as the existence of alternative forms of non-functionalist sociology. He pejoratively characterised these as 'encyclopedism' where sociologists made sweeping claims about their discipline's epistemic jurisdiction and truthfulness; 'reductionism' which sought to explain social phenomena with reference to non-social factors, such as biology, psychology and climate; 'anti-theoretical empiricism' which was content with the description of facts and reporting of statistical relationships; and what might be called 'ethical reformism' where sociologists articulated their own moral values in their work and advocated the reform of society in accordance with them. Davis (1959, 771; emphasis in original) wrote that:

> The early rise of functionalism helped to make a place in sociology and anthropology for those wishing to explain social phenomena in terms of social systems, as against those who wished to make no explanation at all, to explain things in terms of some *other* system, or to plead a cause.

He himself made a major contribution to the development of functionalist sociology by publishing a number of papers on human sexuality prior to or around the beginning of World War II. These papers discussed such topics as jealousy and sexual property, prostitution and illegitimacy (Davis 1936; 1937; 1939a; 1939b). According to Edward Sagarin (1971, 384), in his review of sociological sex research, Davis's work 'constituted the first serious effort (and...the best to date) to understand the nature of sexual mores in terms of social structure, particularly in a functionalist framework.'

Talcott Parsons, however, played the major role in the transition of American sociology toward functionalism (Swingewood 2000, 140). By the end of his 1937 work, *The Structure of Social Action*, he was moving toward a structural-functionalist approach to sociology and this continued in his later work. Many of his major statements on structural-functionalist theory were contained in the works he published in the early 1950s, especially *The Social System* (1951). In this and other works, he focused on how social order was maintained in society. To this end, he analysed the mutually supportive relationships between different social structures which performed positive functions for each other, and which tended to re-establish equilibrium after periods of disturbance. Change itself was seen as a fairly orderly and evolutionary process (Ritzer 1992, 64).

Parsons became the most important exponent of structural-functionalist theory and by the time he published *The Social System* he had become one of the most influential sociologists of his era (Ritzer 1992, 64; Baert 1998, 48). Through the work of Parsons and other functionalist writers, such as Robert Merton, Kingsley Davis and Wilbert Moore, functionalism became the reigning (though not unchallenged) orthodoxy in American sociology in the 1950s and 1960s (Huaco 1986). Kingsley Davis (1959, 771; emphasis in original), in his 1959 Presidential address to the American Sociological Association, even went so far as to argue that 'structural-functional analysis *is* sociological analysis.'

FUNCTIONALIST SOCIOLOGY OF SEX

Functionalism provided some of the first systematic postwar U.S. sociological analysis of sexuality (Stein 1989, 5). It often examined sexuality within the context of the nuclear family and became the 'largest and richest tradition in the sociology of the family' (McIntosh 1987, 144; Stein 1989, 5). Its focus on the family in relation to sex was probably not surprising given the influential psychoanalytic view that sexual behaviour is fundamentally shaped within this institution (Stein 1989, 5). According to Komarovsky and Waller (1945, 448):

> Freudianism may, in fact, be thought of as a sort of familistic social psychology which tends always to explain the behavior of the adult in terms of his previous experience in the parental family and possibly tends to minimize nonfamily and later influences. The Freudian technique is well adapted to the discovery of facets of human behavior which run contrary to the norms of society, such phenomena as infantile sexuality, incestuous attachments, and ambivalence, ...

Functionalists, such as the anthropologist, George Murdock (1949a, 1–2) believed that the nuclear family (typically consisting 'of a married man and woman with their offspring') exists in all societies and is inevitable because it performs certain essential functions for society. In his account, these are sexual, economic, reproductive and educational functions: the sexual and reproductive functions are essential for providing new members of society; the economic function is essential for materially sustaining them; and the educational function is for transmitting knowledge and skills necessary for their ongoing and competent participation in society (Murdock 1949a, 10).

The functionalist view of sexuality was partly influenced by Freud who saw sex and society as antithetical. Sex was believed to be a property of the individual, a powerful biological drive which was very difficult to control and which could pose a threat to the functioning of the social order (Stein 1989, 5; Scanzoni and Marsiglio 1992, 1754). Murdock (1949b, 256), for example, writes that:

> The imperious drive of sex, no less than aggression, is capable of impelling individuals toward behavior disruptive of social relationships. Indiscriminate competition over sexual favors, resulting inevitably in frustrations and jealousies, would impose dangerous strains upon the

fabrics of interpersonal adjustments. Society, therefore, cannot remain indifferent to sex, but must bring it under control.

In some functionalist accounts, male and female sexuality were seen as being biologically different. Males, for example, were seen as having a greater biological impulse for sex, as being more sexually aggressive, and as needing more frequent sexual gratification than females (Pitts 1964, 58). Although individual differences in biologically based sexual traits (e.g. differences in the strength of the sex drive) were believed to exist among members of both sexes, the 'relative uniformity of social behavior is insured... through *cultural and social constraints*....at greater costs, of course, to those human animals on both extremes of the biological range' (Pitts 1964, 59; emphasis in original).

The personal expression of the sex drive was thought to be controllable to some extent by the internalisation (and, if necessary, the enforcement) of appropriate social norms. Functionalists tended to see the nuclear family as the major social institution for controlling sexuality within society, both in terms of regulating adult sexual behaviour, and in reproducing, caring for and socialising children (Davis 1976; Stein 1989, 5; Scanzoni and Marsiglio 1992, 1754).

In relation to the regulation of adult sexual behaviour, Murdock (1949a, 4–5) argues, for example, that the nuclear family performs a sexual function for both its individual members and the wider society. It allows husbands and wives to have the privilege of a sexual relationship and the opportunity to obtain sexual gratification while the norms of society restrict or forbid sexual activity outside marriage. This strengthens the family because the strong emotions associated with sexual activity bind husbands and wives more closely together. Furthermore, the sexual function of marriage helps to maintain social order by restraining the free expression of the sexual impulse. If this impulse was not restrained, then it would press 'individuals to behavior disruptive of the cooperative relationships upon which human social life rests...' (Murdock 1949a, 4).

In relation to the primary socialisation of children, Parsons and Bales (1956, 16), for example, regard this as one of the 'basic and irreducible functions of the family.' Drawing on psychoanalytic theories, and Freud's discussion of psychosexual development, they argue that mothers' (expressive) and fathers' (instrumental) roles need to be clearly distinguished for socialisation to be effective. They see the second 'basic and irreducible' function of the family as stabilising the personalities of the spouses who have to rely on each other to cope with daily life in the relative absence of wider kinship support. They believe this stabilisation can occur through the primary socialisation of children which allows parents to act out the residuary childish aspects of their own personalities which cannot normally be acted out in adult society. Parsons and Bales (1956, 20) regard infantile regression, within limits, as being necessary for a healthy adult personality. They also argue that genital sexuality within marriage has an important regressive (and personality stabilising) function in symbolising for both spouses 'a reenactment of the preoedipal mother-child relationship...' (Parsons and Bales 1956, 21). However, this is seen as being appropriately regulated because sexual love between spouses is usually contingent on them taking 'fully adult responsibilities in roles other than that of marriage directly' (Parsons and Bales 1956, 21–2).

Functionalist accounts of sexuality which adopted a drive model of sexuality from psychoanalysis tended to find uniformity and consistency in the sexual behaviour they studied rather than diversity and behavioural change. 'Heterosexual, procreative sexuality reigned supreme' in their work (Stein 1989, 1). There was one important difference, however, between the psychoanalysts' and the functionalists' views on the effectiveness of the normative control of the sex drive. In the psychoanalytic view, social norms had to be developed to help contain deviant sexual impulses but, at the same time, psychoanalysts tended to assume that the individual's internalisation of such norms would often fail. Functionalists, such as Talcott Parsons, on the other hand, were much more optimistic about the successful internalisation of such norms by social actors. Parsons's concept of the social role — the idea that individuals learn and act in terms of socially defined norms — was based on the assumption that socialisation would usually be effective and that, if not, normative correction of deviance would be relatively straightforward (Stein 1989, 5). Dennis Wrong (1961), however, criticised this 'oversocialised' conception of the individual and argued that socialisation is not the all-powerful process it is often claimed to be.

By the early 1970s, functionalism had lost its pre-eminent theoretical position in U.S. sociology. This was associated with a temporary decline in U.S. world dominance, the social turbulence and radicalism of the 1960s, and criticisms of functionalist thinking which had been mounting since the 1950s. The more general decline of functionalism, and specific criticisms of functionalist studies of sexuality, opened the way for a new sociology of sex — based on a theoretical framework that later came to be known as 'social constructionism'— to emerge in the mid-1970s (Bottomore 1984, 13–14; Huaco 1986; Stein 1989, 6; Vance 1989; Ritzer 1992, 69; Seidman 1994a, 122; Swingewood 2000, 157). 'Social constructionism' is discussed in more detail in chapter 3.

WHY HAVE SOCIOLOGISTS MISUNDERSTOOD THE HISTORY OF THEIR DISCIPLINE'S SEX RESEARCH?

In the preceding section, I argued that there is a sizeable and diverse sociological literature on sex that stretches from at least the 1840s to 1960. Sex has usually had an important role in human affairs, not least because of its role in reproduction, and it would indeed be remarkable if sociologists had ignored the topic to the extent that some writers claim. Given the existence of this literature, then, why have most sociological writers on sex claimed that the sociology of sex did not emerge until the 'postwar era' and as late as the 1960s or 1970s?

An important article by R.W. Connell (1997) provides ideas which help to answer this question. Connell himself is not primarily concerned with this question or answer in his article. He is mainly concerned with the question 'Why is Classical [sociological] Theory Classical?' Nevertheless, in the course of answering his own question, his main arguments and brief comments about the sociological study of sex are very helpful in considering why sociologists might have misunderstood their discipline's history of sex research. One of his main arguments is that the rise and influence of the classical canon in sociology strongly affected how sociologists viewed their discipline and its history.

I pointed out earlier that the process of canon making began in the 1930s in the United States, and was an attempt to reconstruct sociology on more secure foundations after the failure of the evolutionist and empiricist projects. It involved the construction of a canonical point of view, the nomination and acceptance of disciplinary founders and the dissemination of their texts (Connell 1997).

After World War II, the process of canon making was facilitated by the development of a mass higher education system in the United States. Graduate sociology programs expanded within this system to provide training for the sociologists who would teach the growing number of students enrolling in sociology courses. A pedagogy based on 'classical' texts developed at this time in sociology graduate programs. These programs and their pedagogy became central to sociology's definition of itself as a profession (Connell 1997, 1537–8). Eventually the canon was extended to undergraduate sociological curricula, and students, through books of readings in sociological theory which contained extracts from the 'classical' texts. Familiarity with the canon even became required through the Graduate Record Examination (Connell 1997, 1543). Connell (1997, 1540) argues that, by the early 1960s, the canonical view of sociology's history — that sociology was founded by a small group of brilliant intellectuals seeking to understand social changes internal to European and North American societies — had become hegemonic within U.S. sociology. 'The construction of the canon provided not only an intellectual but also a symbolic solution to the internal disintegration and cultural marginalization that had overtaken sociology before the midcentury' (Connell 1997, 1540–1).

In the 1950s and 1960s, during the Cold War, wealthy U.S. foundations helped to fund the export of U.S. sociology abroad. Sociological perspectives, research methods, research problems, textbooks, and even sociologists themselves were exported from the United States to many other places — including Australia, France, Germany, Japan, New Zealand and Scandinavia — where sociology was being established or reconstituted in expanding systems of higher education (Cohn-Bendit, Duteuil, Gerard and Granautier 1969, 375; Connell 1997, 1544). The pedagogy of the canon was exported too. Students in many and varied countries found themselves studying the canonical view of the discipline's history and the classical texts 'as the basic definition of "theory"' (Connell 1997, 1544). Irving Zeitlin (1984, 4) undoubtedly spoke for many sociologists when he stressed the centrality of the classics for the teaching of sociology:

> The essentials of the sociological approach are best conveyed by intro-
> ducing the student to the pioneers of sociological theory and analysis
> who wrote in the late nineteenth and early twentieth centuries. Their
> works are now regarded as the classic tradition of sociological think-
> ing because they have stood the test of time. We refer to these writ-
> ings again and again; we rely on pioneers' theoretical ideas; we employ
> their concepts; we continue to investigate questions they raised; and,
> finally, we emulate their intellectual craftsmanship. In a word, the clas-
> sic tradition provides the theoretical foundations of the sociological
> perspective.

Sociologists also came to identify themselves and their work in terms of particular canonical figures and perspectives. On a global scale, the canon performed the same function it had in U.S. sociology: it provided sociologists and their students with a shared sense of their discipline's core and legitimacy, a set of distinctive symbols, 'a shared language, and some kind of [disciplinary] identity...' (Connell 1997, 1544).

Despite the various functions that the canon has performed for sociology, Connell (1997) argues that they came at a considerable cost. In relation to the question of why most sociological writers on sex did not see a sociology of sex emerging until the 'postwar era', or as late as the 1960s or 1970s, four main points can be made. Firstly, the canonical view of sociology's history 'replaced earlier and very different accounts of the making of sociology' (Connell 1997, 1545). It concealed much of the discipline's history from sociologists, especially the way in which sociology was shaped by, and developed within the social relations of imperialism. The deletion of the discourse of imperialism from sociology meant that the texts which were most explicitly concerned with 'the primitive, the concept of progress, racial hierarchies, and gender and population issues failed to be canonized' (Connell 1997, 1545). In this process, issues such as sexuality, gender and 'race' which were central to evolutionary sociology were marginalised within the discipline. In some cases, canonical authors did discuss these issues in their texts but Connell (1997, 1545) points out that, if they did, then these texts were the least likely to be canonised or used in teaching students. This had the effect of keeping these issues to the margins of the discipline. Even such a supposedly authoritative source on sociology as Oxford University Press's *A Dictionary of Sociology* could claim in 1998, for example, that 'None of the major figures in the discipline [sociology] seems to have attached any importance to the topic [of sexuality] as an area for research or analysis' (Marshall 1998, 595). Similarly, the *International Encyclopedia of the Social & Behavioral Sciences,* claimed in 2001 that the sociology of sexuality only 'emerged in the 1960s and 1970s ...' (Richardson 2001, 14018). Yet, as previously discussed, even canonical authors, such as Marx, Comte, Spencer, Durkheim, Weber and Simmel, among others, did attach at least some importance — and sometimes a lot of importance — to sexuality, and did research and analyse it, even if it was not always in ways which would be approved or accepted today. In 2005, a new online edition of the Oxford dictionary above repeated its earlier view about the major figures in sociology. However, by now it had at least acknowledged that '...Georg Simmel produced some important essays' on sexuality (Scott and Marshall 2005). As Connell (1997, 1515–16) points out more generally about evidence which disconfirms the canon: 'This evidence is unfamiliar because of the canon itself. Most sociologists today do not read early sociological texts *except* the canonical ones' (emphasis in original).

In fact, there have been remarkably few attempts by sociologists to document the research efforts they have undertaken to confirm the supposed absence of a sociological literature on sex. The research which exists is scanty, unsystematic and selective, and often relates to a period when the canon was already hegemonic in sociology (see, for example, Reiss 1967, 2; Plummer 1975, 203; and Seidman 1994b, 168). Plummer (1975, 203) is one of the few sociologists to have attempted this kind of research, and he correctly pointed out that 'The neglect of sociological perspectives on sexuality needs fuller documentation....'

Some of the existing research is also based on invalid indicators. Seidman (1994b, 168), for example, claims that one of the indicators of the lack of sociological research on sexuality is that the index of the *American Journal of Sociology* only lists thirteen articles published on 'sex' between 1895 and 1965. However, there are two main problems with this evidence. Firstly, Seidman's (1994b, 168) figures are wrong. The index shows that there are thirteen *authors* of articles on 'sex' but *fifteen* articles on the topic. Secondly, and more importantly, the index includes articles which are *not* on sexuality under the heading of 'sex' (which Seidman (1994b, 168) acknowledges), such as articles on gender and sex differences; but it also includes articles which are concerned with sexuality under other headings in the index, such as 'Prostitution' 'Incest taboo,' 'Family' and 'Courtship' (Blau 1966) which Seidman seems unaware of. A simple reliance on the number of entries listed under the heading of 'sex' in this index is a poor way of gauging how many articles were published about sexuality in the *American Journal of Sociology* between 1895 and 1965.

The influence of the classical canon probably explains why so few sociologists have bothered to provide any evidence of research which demonstrates an absent sociological literature on sex, and why such research is so cursory and piecemeal. Sociologists who were educated via the pedagogy of the canon (and its story of sociology's origins) would have 'known' that sociologists rarely or never studied sex. Since they already 'knew' this, and this was a common view within their discipline, they probably saw little need to provide evidence for something widely regarded as both true and obvious.

The second point about the relationship between the rise of the classical canon and sociologists' views of their discipline's neglect of sex research is that the rise of the canon changed sociologists' conceptions of sociology. Prior to the process of canon making, there were many different kinds of sociology, including the strands that Davis (1959) identified as encyclope-dism, reductionism, anti-theoretical empiricism, and what might be called ethical reformism. There were debates (some of which continue today) about what sociology is, whether it deserved to exist, whether it is a science, and, if so, what kind of science it is. Its 'areas of study were not at all clearly circumscribed....' and there were many differences of opinion on these issues (Sagarin 1971, 382; Connell 1997, 1536–7).

The rise of the classical canon did not do away with disagreements among sociologists or with different kinds of sociology but it did produce a narrower conception of sociology, and particularly sociological theory, as compared with the past. The classical texts came to symbolise the essence of sociology and would influence what kind of discourses would count as sociological theory (Connell 1997, 1512). This is important to keep in mind when reviewing sociologists' claims about the lack of sex research in sociology's history. Sociologists, such as Sagarin (1971) and Plummer (1975), for example, were clearly aware of some of the early sociological sex research which I have previously mentioned in this chapter. However, from their vantage point in the 1970s, they no longer accepted much of it as sociological. Sagarin (1971, 382) and Plummer (1975, 3), for example, redefined the work of Edward Westermarck and William Graham Sumner (both sociologists whose work was once regarded as sociological) as anthropological. Similarly, they redefined the work of W. I. Thomas (another sociologist) as non-sociological, and, in particular, as anthropological and/or psychological (Sagarin 1971, 383; Plummer 1975, 3). Plummer (1975, 3) suggested that these early 'sociologists' were not really doing sociological work because they explored sexuality 'from viewpoints divorced from sociology.' Sagarin (1971, 382) makes this point clearer when he says that 'many sociologists were deeply immersed in cross-cultural... studies' but, by doing cross-cultural research, he thinks they were really doing anthropology. Both Sagarin (1971) and Plummer (1975) apparently overlooked the fact that cross-cultural studies were once the hallmark of sociology, and particularly evolutionary sociology, during or close to the time when Westermarck, Sumner and Thomas were writing (Connell 1997).

Plummer (1975, 3–4) also denied the label of sociology to other sociological studies of sex. He discounted the sociological aspects of Reich's and Marcuse's work in referring to them as 'essentially metatheoretical excursions...' (Plummer 1975, 3). He also classified the studies by Schofield, Gorer, Dickinson and others 'as social surveys and not sociology' (Plummer 1975, 3). Yet, much of this social survey research belonged to the strand of sociology that Davis (1959) called 'anti-theoretical empiricism.' Davis (1959) was opposed to this kind of sociology but he did not deny that it was regarded as sociology. Similarly, Ehrmann (1963, 142–5) commented that this kind of survey research often used a 'sociological frame of reference' and studied the social determinants of sexual behaviour. Plummer (1975, 3) acknowledged that these are the studies 'most frequently tagged "sociology"'. Yet, he stated that 'Most of the studies commonly regarded as sociological simply do not meet the criteria of that discipline' (Plummer 1975, 3). According to him, this was because the authors of these studies 'have rarely been sociologists interested in theory and working in sociological contexts' (Plummer 1975, 3). In other words, Plummer (1975) seemed to believe that the criteria which he (and others) used to define sociology superseded earlier criteria used to define sociological work.

Sagarin (1971) and Plummer (1975), in fact, were not primarily interested in trying to understand previous sociological work in terms of earlier disciplinary criteria and meanings. Instead, their main concern was to argue for its exclusion from sociology altogether. Furthermore, they never explicitly spelt out their own criteria for defining sociology even though they markedly agreed on what counted and did not count as sociology. It seems likely that their common position was a reflection of what accorded with the canonical view of sociology which had long been hegemonic within the discipline at the time they were writing. This is difficult to prove conclusively due to the lack of detail they give about their disciplinary criteria. However, their lack of detail on, or even defence of, their criteria may itself be an indication that they expected this criteria to be well understood and accepted by their sociological peers. This expectation, in turn, was very likely because the criteria itself was part of, and conformed to, the canonical view of sociology which by now had become part of sociological common sense.

There are also other indications that the canonical view may have influenced Sagarin's (1971) and Plummer's (1975) views of sociology and what they counted as belonging to the discipline. Sagarin (1971, 382–3), for example, thought it ironic that early sociologists did not study the sexuality of 'modern societies and especially... their own' when they were studying these societies, particularly at the macro level, in terms of 'social structure, class, institutions, power, and groups, in which sexuality seemed to play little or no role.' This certainly conforms with the canonical view of sociology's history which incorrectly emphasises how early sociologists focused most of their attention on social changes internal to European and North American societies. Similarly, Plummer (1975, 3) commented that sociologists have to be 'interested in theory' for their work to be counted as sociological. He does not say what he means by 'theory' but, as Connell (1997, 1512) points out, the rise of the classical canon came to define what 'counts as sociological theory.' The research which Plummer (1975, 3) wanted to exclude from sociology seems inconsistent with this later conception of theory but, in any case, his emphasis on theory excluded the atheoretical empiricist work which was once regarded as sociology.

The main implications of this canonical revisionism of the sociology of sex are that the history of sociology is misrepresented; the history of sociological sex research is interpreted as being more meagre and less diverse than it actually is; and the traditions of sex research in other disciplines, such as anthropology and psychology, are bolstered by the reassignment of formerly sociological sex research to new disciplinary homes.

The third point about the influence of the classical canon on sociology is that it did not just affect how sociologists understood the history of their discipline or their conception of sociology. It also affected many sociologists' conceptions of the topics or 'problems' that sociology should be concerned with as a discipline (Connell 1997, 1545–6). The remaking of sociology's history in terms of the canon gave many sociologists a sense that because the canonical texts did not deal very much with topics like sexuality, 'race' and gender, that these topics were also unimportant for contemporary sociology. In effect, the process of canon making narrowed sociology's intellectual scope by excluding and discrediting what was not canonical.

There is certainly some evidence from both the United States and Britain that, at the time when the canon was hegemonic within sociology, relatively few sociologists were showing significant interest in and/or conducting sex research (see, for example, Reiss 1967, 2; Krausz 1969; Collison and Webber, 1971; and Plummer 1975, 203; although they do not interpret the evidence in these terms). Even as late as 1994, a supposedly authoritative source on sociology, such as *The Penguin Dictionary of Sociology* had no major entry on 'Sex' or 'Sexuality' within its pages. The authors of the dictionary stated that 'A dictionary of sociology is not just a collection of definitions, but inevitably a statement of what the discipline is' (Abercrombie et al 1994, vii). By their own account, then, the authors of this dictionary must have held the view that sex and sexuality had no place within sociology and were completely irrelevant to the discipline. Since the authors also claimed that their book was 'prescriptive in suggesting lines of development and consolidation' in the discipline, it is even more surprising that they apparently did not even see sex and sexuality as topics on the horizon (Abercrombie et al 1994, vii). The closest alphabetical listings to these topics in the dictionary were 'Sexism' and 'Sexual Divisions' (Abercrombie et al 1994, 375). By the year 2000, *The Penguin Dictionary of Sociology* had finally and very belatedly included an entry on 'sexualities'. It made the astounding claim that while sociology had traditionally distinguished between 'sex' and 'gender', 'More recently, sociologists have also identified sexuality as the mode by which sexual interest and sexual preference are expressed' (Abercrombie et al 2000, 313). This seems to suggest that sociologists have only discovered or taken an interest in these matters at the virtual turn of the millennium. Connell (1997, 1546) points out that:

> The continuing influence of the canon in defining what counts is one of the main reasons why gender and race, though now institutionally important for American sociology (as shown by affirmative action programs or the sections of the ASA [American Sociological Association], have still not reestablished themselves as central concerns of sociological theory.

A similar point can be made about sexuality. The continuing influence of the canon in sociology is undoubtedly a major reason why sexuality has not reestablished itself as a central concern of sociological theory and why it did not become 'institutionalised as a formal subfield of sociological study' (Epstein 1994, 188; see also Connell and Dowsett 1992, 49; Irvine 1994, 233; and Laumann and Gagnon 1995, 184). Furthermore, 'few sociologists participate in the burgeoning interdisciplinary field of sexuality studies,' and while there are important exceptions, '[M]uch of this work is recent' (Irvine 1994, 233; Nagel 2000, 109; Gamson and Moon 2004, 48).

The canonical view of sociology's disciplinary boundaries, however, is not the only or even the best view available. An alternative position would be to argue that sociology must, in some sense, be commensurate with the ontological features of the object under study: for example, human society (Sharp, R. 2001, pers. comm. 4 September; Lawson 1997, 34–5; Archer 1998, 194). This is because what sociology can know about that object, and how sociology can study it, will partly depend on the nature of the object itself (as well as a range of other factors). For example, if social structures depend on intentional human agency, then some understanding of this agency will need to be a part of the discipline. Similarly, if society is inherently dynamic, then sociology will need to develop theoretical perspectives and methods which enable this to be properly understood (Lawson 1997, 34–5).

If sociology is concerned with the study of human sexuality within society, then, again, the sociology of sex or sexuality must, in some way, be commensurate with the social dimensions of this object. For example, it could be argued that sociology needs to be concerned with at least two broad issues here: firstly, how sexuality is socially defined; and secondly, how the various phenomena which fall under this definition are caused, or constituted by the 'social', how they affect the 'social', and how they are interpreted and understood in terms of it. In trying to understand the relevant aspects of its particular object, sociology may also have to take some cognisance of the way in which this object can be studied in interrelated ways by other scientific disciplines, such as biology and psychology

(Mahoney 1983, ch. 2). This might mean that sociology, at times, has to revise its own ideas of its object of study as a result of its own research or the research of other sciences. This could obviously have implications for the way that disciplinary or subdisciplinary boundaries are drawn in sociology at particular times. While this chapter has argued that the disciplinary boundaries of sociology have narrowed for historical reasons during the twentieth century, the ontological features of the object under study must not be neglected if sociology is to do justice both to itself and its subject matter.

Finally, the sociologists who believed that the sociology of sex first developed in the 1960s or early 1970s were noticing something important within the discipline even if they misinterpreted its meaning. From the mid-1960s on, perspectives and studies of sexuality based on aspects of the Freudian tradition, comparative sociology, the sociology of deviance, symbolic interactionism and labelling theory began to gain momentum in sociology (Plummer 1982, 226; Vance 1991, 876). Important published works included those by McIntosh (1992 [1968]), Henslin (1971), Gagnon and Simon (1973), Plummer (1975) and Gagnon (1977). This was not the beginning of a sociology of sex, as some people claimed, but it did break with much of the earlier sociology of sex. It opened up new questions and insights on sexuality (despite its own limitations), and it was an important forerunner and influence on social construction theory which developed in the mid-1970s (Plummer 1982; Simon and Gagnon 1986, 104; Vance 1991, 876; Schneider and Nardi 1999; Gamson and Moon 2004).

SOCIOLOGICAL RESPONSES TO MASTERS AND JOHNSON

Shortly after the canon had become hegemonic in U.S. sociology, and while functionalism still dominated that branch of the discipline, Masters and Johnson published their major works, *Human Sexual Response* (1966) and *Human Sexual Inadequacy* (1970). These works were widely and positively reviewed and greeted with great acclaim ('Playboy Interview: Masters and Johnson' 1976; Zilbergeld and Evans 1980). Sociologists[1] were undoubtedly aware of the popular reaction to these publications but they have largely ignored the study and analysis of these works since they were published. When they did mention them it was often to include their content in textbooks on human sexuality concerning human sexual response and sex therapy (see, for example, Gochros and Schultz 1972; Gagnon 1977) or to

---

1. I am using a wide definition of 'sociologist' here to include those who study and write about sexuality from sociological perspectives even if they identify their disciplinary or institutional locations in terms of some other academic specialisation, such as psychiatry or psychology.

favourably compare Masters and Johnson's work with earlier sex research and methods of treating sexual dysfunctions (see, for example, Koedt 1973; Lo Piccolo and Heiman 1977). Sociologists often accepted — at little more than face value — Masters and Johnson's (1966) claims that they provided objective scientific data about the physiology of human sexual response and that they had dispelled harmful myths about human sexuality (see, for example, Lo Piccolo and Heiman 1977; Gagnon 1977; and Leiblum and Pervin 1980). As Laws and Schwartz (1977, vii) put it:

> By bringing sexual behavior into the laboratory for study, Masters and Johnson set a new standard for evidence in theories about sex. This was a departure from the research tradition that until that time had relied only on uncorroborated reports of past events obtained from sources such as interviews or questionnaires. In the laboratory, stimulation could be controlled and responses measured objectively; findings could be replicated.

Sociologists also credited the success of Masters and Johnson's (1966) research with helping to break down some of the barriers to sex research for sociologists and other researchers (Sagarin 1971, 393; Gagnon 1977, 134–5). According to Sagarin (1971, 393):

> the generally favourable reception of this work [*Human Sexual Response*], the high esteem in which it was held, and the ability to withstand the criticism of it on ethical grounds meant that no holds were barred in sex research. The influence of this study on sociological investigation is quite readily understandable.... Masters and Johnson, investigating at a university, publishing in scientific journals, proved as formidable in the removal of barriers to sex research as had Freud and Kinsey before them.

In some cases, sociologists made minor criticisms of Masters and Johnson's (1966) research and added qualifications to the interpretation of their findings. Gagnon (1977, 131), for example, pointed out that Masters and Johnson provided 'no extended discussion' of their charts depicting male and female sexual response nor of their charts' meaning. He also explained how Masters and Johnson's descriptions of human sexual response were only approximations of aspects of sexual response and that they could not be completely generalised to people's sexual responses outside the laboratory (Gagnon 1977, 134). However, sociologists in the 1970s seem to have been largely unaware of, or ignored, the existence of more significant criticisms of Masters and Johnson's (1966) research by the philosopher Irving Singer (1973) and the historian Paul Robinson (1976).

It was a similar story with the publication of *Human Sexual Inadequacy* in 1970. Sociologists largely accepted Masters and Johnson's (1970) claims about their sex therapy at face value. For example, sociologists tended to regard Masters and Johnson as having developed a new approach to understanding and treating sexual dysfunctions which was astonishingly successful. They subjected Masters and Johnson's (1970) claims to very little probing or analysis (see, for example, Lo Piccolo and Heiman 1977; Gagnon 1977; Leiblum and Pervin 1980).

Some sociologists even wanted to join Masters and Johnson's sex therapy 'revolution.' After Masters and Johnson (1970) wrote about the role of social factors in sexual dysfunction, some clinical sociologists saw new vocational and business opportunities for themselves as sociological sex educators. The aim of this sex education was to prevent or cure sexual dysfunctions in their clients and students (Lavender 1985).

When sociologists did criticise Masters and Johnson's (1970) research, the criticisms mainly consisted of questioning the concept of sexual dysfunction; identifying populations which might not benefit from Masters and Johnson's type of therapy; and pointing out how the dissemination of Masters and Johnson's research findings contributed (against the sex researchers' own intentions) to new performance pressures on people to have sex in the scientifically approved way (Lo Piccolo and Heiman 1977; Gagnon 1977; Leiblum and Pervin 1980).

In 1980, two major critiques of Masters and Johnson's (1966; 1970) work were published which contributed to scepticism about their scientific and clinical claims. The first was by the psychologists, Zilbergeld and Evans (1980). They systematically challenged Masters and Johnson's (1970) reporting of treatment outcome statistics and the effectiveness of their sex therapy program. (This critique is discussed in more detail in chapter 7). The other major critique was by the psychiatrist Thomas Szasz. In his book *Sex By Prescription* (1980) (published in Britain in 1981 as *Sex: Facts, Frauds and Follies*), Szasz (1981, xii) argued that '"Scientific" sexology is a veritable Trojan horse: appearing to be modernity's gift to mankind in its struggle for freedom and dignity, it is, in fact, just another strategy for its pacification and enslavement.'

In his book, Szasz (1981) questioned many of the basic assumptions underpinning sex research, sex therapy and sex education. For example, he questioned medical conceptions of 'sick' sexual behaviour; the legitimacy of clinicians in defining and treating such behaviour; the objectivity and value freedom of sex research; the hidden moral and political basis of sex therapy (which largely concerned Masters and Johnson's work); and the legitimacy and accuracy of contemporary sex education.

Szasz's critique shook the intellectual foundations of scientific sexology. In 1981, the Society for the Scientific Study of sex acknowledged the force of Szasz's critique by inviting him to outline his position at the plenary session of its annual conference before 400 professional sexologists. Szasz (1983) obliged with a paper subsequently published as 'Speaking about sex: Sexual pathology and sexual therapy as rhetoric.' The Society for the

Scientific Study of Sex also invited four eminent sexologists — Erwin Haeberle, Joseph Lo Piccolo, Mary Calderone and John Gagnon — to reply to Szasz's (1981; 1983) position. The responses ranged from those which accepted Szasz's basic concerns but saw his attack on Masters and Johnson as 'rather misguided' (Haeberle 1983); to those which acknowledged the valuable service Szasz's critique provided to sexology even if they disagreed with many of his individual points (Lo Piccolo 1983); to those which did not directly respond to Szasz but which provided their own views of basic sexological issues, such as education for sexuality (Calderone 1983); and, finally, those which attempted to understand Szasz's criticisms in relation to broader social and historical changes affecting the nature of sexuality, on the one hand, and sex research, education and therapy on the other (Gagnon 1983). The main papers in this dispute were collected together and published in an edited volume entitled *Challenges in Sexual Science*. The editor, Clive Davis (1983, iii), frankly acknowledged in his preface to the book that Szasz had 'called into question the basic assumptions... directing our sex research, sex education, and sex therapy', and that the theoretical foundations of sexology were inadequate.

Following Szasz's (1981) critique, a small number of sociological books and journal articles were published in the 1980s which focused on selected aspects of Masters and Johnson's (1966, 1970) work and its social consequences. Feminist analyses focused on the relationship between Masters and Johnson's (1966) research, feminism and the sexual revolution (Ehrenreich, Hess and Jacobs 1987, ch. 2); the way in which sexologists, including Masters and Johnson, supported models of male sexuality and heterosexuality which reinforced male supremacy over women (Jackson 1984a); and the way in which sex therapy ignored the social aspects of women's sexual problems and reinforced gender inequality (Seidler-Feller 1985). Other sociological research concerning Masters and Johnson's (1966; 1970) work, in the 1980s, focused on criticisms of Masters and Johnson's findings on human sexual response and some aspects of their classification of sexual dysfunction (Mahoney 1983); analysis of how Masters and Johnson triumphed over psychoanalysis in the market for sex therapy services (Bejin 1986a); and accounts of how the growing influence of rational sexology brought questionable benefits for people's sex lives (Bejin 1986b).

From 1990 until the turn of the millennium there were probably only five main sociological studies of Masters and Johnson's (1966; 1970) work published. Irvine's (1990a) important feminist study of U.S. sexology, *Disorders of Desire*, devoted a chapter to critically discussing the background, context, nature, consequences and limitations of Masters and Johnson's sex research, and about a third of a chapter to discussing similar issues in regard to their sex therapy program. Tiefer (1991b) published a ground breaking critique of Masters and Johnson in a journal article which focused on historical, scientific, clinical and feminist criticisms of their model of the human sexual response cycle. Boyle (1994) criticised aspects of Masters and

Johnson's (1970) classification of sexual dysfunction and their therapeutic program. This was part of a broader article on 'expert' constructions of sexual problems in the twentieth century. In 1994, I published a critique of the sexological construction of sexual dysfunction and of sexology as an institution of social control (Morrow 1994). This focused primarily on Masters and Johnson's work. I also published a specific critique of Masters and Johnson's concept and classification of sexual dysfunction (Morrow 1996). Other sociological studies in this period which contained important insights into, and criticisms of, Masters and Johnson's (1966; 1970) work included those by Irvine (1990b); Jeffreys (1990); Reiss (1990); Connell and Dowsett (1992); Gardetto (1992); and Boyle (1993).

In sum, then, although sociologists have not completely ignored Masters and Johnson, there has been very little sociological analysis or critique of their work in the forty or so years since *Human Sexual Response* was first published. The analysis and critique which does exist is contained in a small number of book chapters and journal articles (and even sections of chapters and articles) few of which are either solely or predominantly concerned with Masters and Johnson's (1966; 1970) research. Furthermore, the analyses of Masters and Johnson are primarily focused on select and discrete components of their work, such as their model of the human sexual response cycle (Tiefer 1991b), their concept and classification of sexual dysfunction (Morrow 1996) or their competition with psychoanalysis for the sex therapy market (Bejin 1986a). Many of these analyses have also been non-cumulative in the sense that their authors have not cited (and perhaps have been unaware of) important earlier studies which were relevant to their own research. For example, Bejin (1986a; 1986b) wrote about Masters and Johnson's (1970) sex therapy program without referring to the important and relevant work of Szasz (1981) or Zilbergeld and Evans (1980). Tiefer's (1991b) critique of Masters and Johnson's (1966) model of the human sexual response cycle made no reference to the work of Singer (1973) who had anticipated some of her criticisms. And my own first article on Masters and Johnson (Morrow 1994) was written without knowing about relevant earlier studies by Tiefer (1991b) and Irvine (1990a).

To date, there has been no major sociological attempt to provide a book-length analysis or critique of Masters and Johnson's (1966; 1970) work by integrating original analysis of their main texts with the findings of an extensive critical review of their work. The main sociological work on Masters and Johnson is probably Janice Irvine's (1990a) *Disorders of Desire*. Yet her aims are different from those described above. Her study is not primarily about Masters and Johnson. She devotes less than one and a half chapters of her book to their sexual physiology research and sex therapy program. This, along with other topics in her book, is subsumed within the broader theme of 'Sex and Gender in Modern American Sexology' (the subtitle and main theme of her work) (Irvine 1990a). In addition, her literature review on Masters and Johnson, while broad and suitable for her own particular purpose, has a number of important omissions. For example, her study does not take into account some of the earlier but important scholarly sources on Masters and Johnson, such as Szasz (1981), Mahoney (1983) and Bejin (1986a). Her work has also been partly overtaken by some of the newer analyses of Masters and Johnson which were published during the 1990s (see, for example, the work by Tiefer 1991b; Boyle 1994; and Morrow 1996). Irvine (2005) published a revised and expanded edition of *Disorders of Desire* in 2005 but it contains no substantial new material on Masters and Johnson.

WHY HAVE SOCIOLOGISTS LARGELY IGNORED THE STUDY AND ANALYSIS OF MASTERS AND JOHNSON'S (1966; 1970) WORK?

Given that the existing sociological literature on Masters and Johnson's (1966; 1970) research is small, sparse, and often non-cumulative, why have sociologists largely ignored the investigation and analysis of their work? It should be clear already, from the preceding discussion in this chapter, that the sociological neglect of Masters and Johnson's research cannot be adequately explained in terms of the social repression of sexuality which is supposed to have almost completely stifled sociological research on sexuality until the 1960s or 1970s. This chapter has already documented some of the main contours of sociological sex research, particularly in the United States, up to 1960, and explained the lack of awareness of this research among many sociologists in terms of the influence of the classical canon. Nor can the lack of sociological analysis of Masters and Johnson be explained by arguing that the sociology of sex was incapable of providing such analysis because it was newly born at the time when Masters and Johnson's work was published. This chapter has established that sociological study and writing about sexuality long predated the publication of *Human Sexual Response* in 1966, and can be found at least as far back as the 1840s.

Why, then, have sociologists largely neglected Masters and Johnson? There seem to be three main reasons. Firstly, the rise of the classical canon in sociology seems responsible for much of the general neglect of sex research by sociologists. The canon had become hegemonic within U.S .sociology by the early 1960s (before the publication of Masters and Johnson's 1966; 1970 work) and was extending and embedding itself within the knowledge base and pedagogy of sociology in many other countries (Connell 1997). As previously discussed, the canon largely deleted sexuality from dominant conceptions of sociology, from the discipline's history, and from the list of topics regarded as worthy of sociological study. Around the time that Masters and Johnson's (1966; 1970) work was published, relatively few sociologists in Britain or the United States were showing significant interest in and/or conducting sex research, and sexuality was marginal to the main concerns of the discipline. This situation had not greatly changed even by the 1990s (Reiss 1967, 2; Krausz 1969; Collison and Webber 1971; Plummer 1975, 203; Irvine 1994, 233; Laumann and Gagnon 1995, 184).

The hegemony of the canon helps to account for a lower level of sex research by sociologists than probably would have been the case if that hegemony did not exist. However, the hegemony of the canon did not completely prevent sociological sex research. In the time since Masters and Johnson's research was first published, sociologists have studied sexuality across a wide range of substantive areas, using a variety of theoretical perspectives and almost every conceivable and relevant kind of research method (McKinney 1986; Geer and O'Donohue 1987; Weinberg 1994, 564–7). Yet, as discussed above, very little of even this marginal sociological sex research was concerned with Masters and Johnson's research and therapy. This means that other factors were also important in accounting for the sociological neglect of these researchers.

A second reason for the dearth of sociological research on Masters and Johnson's (1966; 1970) work has to do with the hegemonic biomedical and clinical definitions of their work. Masters and Johnson (1966) were working within the biomedical tradition of sex research where sex was conceptualised as a natural biological function rooted in the needs and imperatives of an evolving species (Gagnon and Simon 1973, 4). In their first book, *Human Sexual Response*, for example, Masters and Johnson were primarily concerned with the anatomy and physiology of human sexual functioning. The hegemony of the biomedical view of sex and Masters and Johnson's restricted focus on sexual physiology were major impediments to a sociological understanding of these issues (Epstein 1994, 189–90). Gagnon and Simon (1973, 5), for example, pointed out that:

> Rarely do we turn from a consideration of the organs themselves to the sources of the meanings that are attached to them, the ways in which the physical activities of sex are learned, and the ways in which these activities are integrated into larger social scripts and social arrangements where meaning and sexual behavior come together to create sexual conduct.

At the same time, the laboratory setting of Masters and Johnson's research and their methods of investigation had little relevance to most sociological research on sexuality (McKinney 1986, 115).

It was a similar story with Masters and Johnson's (1970) second book, *Human Sexual Inadequacy*. It was concerned with treating sexually dysfunctional couples, classifying sexual dysfunctions, explaining their aetiology, outlining the principles of their sex therapy program, and evaluating its effectiveness. This sort of work was also part of the clinical/medical tradition of sex research where doctors and clinicians undertook sex research

because they were being consulted by patients experiencing sexual problems of one kind or another (Gebhard 1968, 395; Sagarin 1968, 2). Within
this tradition, people's sexual problems were mostly regarded as personal
problems. This meant they were usually understood in idiosyncratic ways
rather than in terms of a sociological framework. These problems were
also believed to be solvable, if they were solvable, through therapy which
was the domain of the doctor, psychiatrist or psychologist (Sagarin 1971,
384; Haeberle 1980, 70). 'The emphasis on pathology by psychologists,
psychiatrists and medical doctors helps to legitimize their investigations'
(Reiss 1967, 2). Perhaps because sociologists lacked these kinds of medical and therapeutic legitimations (or alternative defensible legitimations),
they were rarely concerned with this field of research and practice (Sagarin
1971, 385; McKinney 1986, 113). One of the consequences was that little
was 'written on the resolution of practical sexual problems through either
social policy or interpersonal intervention...' (Plummer 1975, 203).

The third reason for the sociological neglect of Masters and Johnson is
probably due to the perceived high quality and importance of their scientific and clinical work. Their scientific research was generally accepted as
ground breaking, and was regarded by, perhaps, most people as careful,
rigorous, dispassionate, objective and convincing. The main debate about
Masters and Johnson's research on human sexual response concerned the
ethics of directly studying people having sex rather than the objectivity of
their findings. Furthermore, this was a debate which Masters, Johnson and
their supporters won. Similarly, the development of their sex therapy program was generally seen as long overdue, and their treatment regarded as
sound and highly effective. There were few obvious signs that Masters and
Johnson were presenting ideology rather than science in their sex research
or that their sex therapy program had important limitations and questionable consequences. Had there been such signs, the sociological response
might well have been different (Guttmacher 1970; Belliveau and Richter
1971, 64; Sagarin 1971, 393; Suggs and Marshall 1971, 222; Beaton Peterson and Peterson 1973; 'Playboy Interview: Masters and Johnson' 1976,
131; Zilbergeld and Evans 1980, 30; Goettsch 1987).

When sociological critiques of Masters and Johnson's (1966; 1970)
work did emerge, it is, perhaps, not surprising that they generally came
from outside academic sociology. They came from disciplines and fields like
psychiatry (Thomas Szasz), psychology (Leonore Tiefer and Mary Boyle),
education (Margaret Jackson) and sexology (Janice Irvine, although in
Irvine's case sociology did inform her perspective). Furthermore, many of
these critiques came from scholars and clinicians who were themselves trying to understand and treat patients with sexual problems (for example,
Irvine, Tiefer and Boyle) (Davis 1983, x; Boyle 1993, 73; Tiefer 1995, 1–2;
Jackson 1984b, 43; Irvine 1990a, Preface; Irvine 2005; Afterword). There
were very few critiques of Masters and Johnson's (1966; 1970) work by

academic or research sociologists (for exceptions, see the work of Bejin 1986a; 1986b; and Morrow 1994; 1996). The impetus for these various critiques came not only from practitioners' clinical experience and radical currents within non-sociology disciplines but also from a variety of other areas, such as conflict theory, symbolic interactionism, social construction theory, feminism, the sociology of deviance, the sociology of knowledge, the sociology of medicine (or the sociology of health and illness), and the sociology of the professions.

Almost all the main sociological critiques of Masters and Johnson's (1966; 1970) work occurred from 1980 and onwards. This was probably due to a confluence of different factors. Four of them seem particularly important. Firstly, Szasz's (1970; 1974) critique of psychiatry and med-icalisation was extended to sex research, sex therapy and sex education in 1980. His critique highlighted many of the inadequacies of sexology and influenced later critiques of Masters and Johnson (see, for example, Seidler-Feller 1985; and Morrow 1994). Secondly, by 1980, sex therapists were realising they could not reproduce Masters and Johnson's (1970) low treatment failure rates, serious doubts were emerging about Masters and Johnson's reporting of treatment outcome statistics, and evidence was mounting that Masters and Johnson's sex therapy program would not be the panacea for sexual dysfunction that they had hoped (Zilbergeld and Evans 1980). Szasz's (1981) critique, and the growing doubts about Mas-ters and Johnson's sex therapy program, prompted further re-examination of the sex researchers' ideas about sexual dysfunction, and their earlier research on human sexual response which had provided them with norms of healthy sexual functioning. Criticisms that were first articulated by writers like Singer (1973) and Robinson (1976) were then rediscovered or developed into more systematic critiques (see, for example, Tiefer 1991b; and Irvine 1990a). Thirdly, the early 1980s was a time when sexuality was re-emerging as an important theoretical issue within feminism. This was after a period in the second half of the 1970s when there was relatively little feminist discussion and writing on this topic (Segal 1983, 31). Some of the most important critiques of Masters and Johnson's work have come from feminist scholars, such as Irvine (1990a), Tiefer (1991b) and Boyle (1994). Finally, social construction theory emerged in the mid-1970s and provided new ways of thinking about and analysing sexuality (Vance 1989; 1991). It has been a major influence on sociological critiques of Masters and John-son from the 1980s onwards.

However, as discussed above, the existing critiques of Masters and Johnson, while important, are relatively few in number. They are typically focused on discrete elements of their work, and are often non-cumulative in the relevant literature. A more systematic analysis and critique is required and this book is intended as a contribution to that end.

CONCLUSION

The research for this chapter developed from the need to understand the sociological response to Masters and Johnson's (1966; 1970) work. In the course of trying to understand that response, and to locate it in relation to previous sociological sex research, it became necessary to examine the history of the sociology of sex. The study of that history led me to reject the conventional view of it that is found in the sociological literature and to offer a new interpretation in this chapter. The discussion of that history is both important in itself and in understanding the sociological response to Masters and Johnson.

The chapter began by introducing and outlining the conventional and taken for granted sociological view about the sociology of sex. According to this view, the sociology of sex was virtually non-existent before World War II and only emerged at some disputed time in the postwar era. The alleged lack of a sociology of sex was 'explained' in various ways but often in terms of a repressive social order which stifled sex research. The alleged emergence of a sociology of sex in the postwar era, and as late as the 1960s or 1970s in some accounts, was also 'explained' by the lessening of social repression and the growing ability of sociologists to grasp the opportunity to study this topic.

This chapter criticised the conventional view and argued that, despite repression, sociology was part of the discursive explosion about sexuality that characterised Western societies from the eighteenth century. The chapter then traced, and discussed at length, some of the main contours and developments in the sociology of sex from the 1840s to 1960, focusing particularly on the United States.

I argued that sociologists have often misunderstood their discipline's history of sex research. This was generally because the rise of the classical canon from the 1930s altered many sociologists' conceptions of sociology, the history of their discipline and the kind of topics that were thought worthy of study. What some sociologists interpreted as the beginning of the sociology of sex in the 1960s or early 1970s was, in fact, a process whereby new perspectives on sexuality gained momentum and visibility within the discipline against more established views.

I then discussed how Masters and Johnson's (1966; 1970) major works were published during a time when the classical canon and functionalism were hegemonic, particularly within U.S. sociology. I noted that sociological responses to Masters and Johnson have mainly come from outside academic sociology; that they have been few in number; that they have been frequently uncritical (particularly the earlier ones from the 1970s); that they have been relatively narrow in their research focus; and that they have often been non-cumulative in the relevant scholarly literature. The lack of sociological attention to Masters and Johnson's work was explained in terms of the influence of the classical canon, the way in which their work was defined in hegemonic biomedical and clinical terms, and the perceived high quality and importance of their work.

I then argued that most of the major sociological critiques of Masters and Johnson's (1966; 1970) work occurred from about 1980 and onwards. This was probably due to the influence of a number of factors including the impact of Szasz's (1981) critique of Masters and Johnson, growing doubts about the effectiveness and treatment outcome statistics of Masters and Johnson's sex therapy program, the re-emergence of sex as an important theoretical issue within feminism, and the rise of social construction theory from the mid-1970s.

Finally, I noted the need for a more systematic sociological analysis and critique of Masters and Johnson's (1966; 1970) work than presently exists. In order to fulfil this aim, it is firstly necessary to discuss some of the major theoretical perspectives on sexuality, and this is the subject of the next chapter.

3 Theoretical Perspectives on Sexuality

INTRODUCTION

The starting point of any sociological research must be with the development of an appropriate and adequate theoretical perspective for studying a selected topic. There are two main theoretical perspectives which have largely influenced thinking about sexuality in Western societies (Connell and Dowsett 1992; DeLamater and Hyde 1998; Harding 1998). The first is usually known as 'essentialism' but is sometimes referred to as 'nativism'. The second perspective is also known under a number of different labels, such as 'social constructionism', 'social constructivism' and 'frame' theories of sexuality. The terms 'essentialism' and 'social constructionism' will be used to denote these theoretical frameworks in this book as these terms are probably the most common and well known of the labels currently in use. This chapter will outline each of these theoretical perspectives, the implications they have for the study and understanding of sexuality, and the major criticisms of them. It will be argued toward the end of the chapter that social constructionism needs to be substantially modified if it is to provide a defensible and useful social science framework for studying sexuality, and for analysing Masters and Johnson's work.

ESSENTIALISM

'Essentialism' is a term which has a variety of different meanings and which designates a number of somewhat different philosophical positions (Keat and Urry 1982, 42–3; Flew 1984, 112; Sayer 1992, 162–4). Perhaps the most important meaning, however, refers to a metaphysical view which can be traced back to Aristotle. Here, essentialism is classically defined as a belief that certain entities have essences which constitute what these entities are. That is, the entities have certain essential or necessary properties 'without which they could not exist or be the things they are' (Flew 1984, 112). The essence of gold, for example, might include the fact that it has the atomic number 79, and the essence of water the fact that it is H20. By contrast, accidental properties are those properties of a thing which are not essential to what it is. For example, gold can exist in the shape of a coin or a ring but the shape itself is accidental to it and not essential. Similarly, it is an accidental property of water as to whether it is found in a glass or in a puddle (Sayer 1997, 456).

Essentialists generally believe that it is important to distinguish between the essential and accidental properties of an entity, or type of entity, and the search for essences has a long history in Western thought. When Socrates, for example, wanted to discover the essence of a phenomenon, such as truth or justice, he wanted a definition which would be true for that phenomenon for all times and places and for nothing else. This meant that the properties discovered had to be essential and not accidental (Blackburn 1996, 125; Martin 1994, 632).

This form of essentialism, however, may be problematic or open to question. Philosophers have long recognised that there are certain metaphysical and epistemological problems associated with the search for essences and that the distinction between essential and accidental properties can be difficult to adequately ground. If, for example, one discovers a property that all members of a particular category, such as woman, have in common, then how is it possible to know whether the property is essential or accidental? In some cases, it might be possible to test or determine what difference the absence of certain properties makes to the entities under consideration (Sayer 1997, 459). In other cases, this might be more difficult. However, if it is decided that a certain property is essential then questions may still remain about its ontological status. Essentialists might claim, for example, that woman's essence is fixed yet actual women alter over time. Woman's essence might also be regarded as eternal yet every woman is mortal. These kinds of examples can raise questions about what kind of thing an essence actually is and how the thing that has an essence is related to particular instances of that thing in the real world (Martin 1994, 632).

ESSENTIALISM AND GENDER

Questions and criticisms of essentialism, however, are by no means only confined to philosophy. As essentialist ideas and assumptions have percolated into other disciplines and fields of inquiry they have taken a variety of forms and drawn their own distinctive responses. In feminist writing, for example, the term 'essentialism' has often been used to denote the view that females or males have their own essential natures (for instance that females are caring, passive and emotional while males are non-caring, active and rational). Differences in these allegedly essential natures have, in turn, frequently been grounded in the separation of mind and body in Western thought so that women's allegedly inferior natures are anchored in their biology while men's allegedly superior natures are tied to the rationality of their non-material minds (Blackburn 1996, 125; Martin 1994, 634). In much essentialist thinking the different natures of men and women which apparently emerge from these dissimilar essences are then used to 'explain' institutionalised patterns of masculine domination and feminine subordination in human societies.

Feminists have often criticised this kind of essentialist thinking on two main grounds. Firstly, the view that, for example, all women have essential natures can produce an illusion of sameness among women. It is often assumed that if all instances of the category woman have a set of common essences then they are alike in all respects. This reasoning is not only invalid but it serves to deny and mask real differences among women. These differences need to be properly taken into account if social research is to grapple with the complexity of women's lives and if effective political action is to be built on a recognition of this complexity (Martin 1994, 636). Secondly, essentialist arguments frequently rely on an ontology 'which stands outside the sphere of cultural influence and historical change' (Fuss 1989, 3). Thus, the idea that men and women have essential natures can be opposed to the view that these 'natures' differ primarily as a result of contingent or accidental factors which are primarily of a sociocultural nature (Blackburn 1996, 125). In fact, it is comparative research, both historical and cross-cultural, which has been most effective in challenging naive essentialist accounts of sex differences in human nature (see, for example, Oakley 1972). And insofar as essentialist accounts of human nature rely on such an ontology to explain social inequalities, they will help to foster the idea that these inequalities are relatively intractable and that sociopolitical action to reduce them will be largely misconceived and ineffective.

ESSENTIALISM AND SEXUALITY

Essentialist assumptions not only characterise certain ways of thinking about gender and gender inequality, they are also clearly evident in the closely related field of sexuality. Essentialism is, in fact, the dominant (though not unchallenged) way of thinking about sexuality in Western societies. It is so pervasive that most people in these societies grow up learning to think about sexuality in essentialist terms without realising that it is a particular perspective and that it is not the only view of sexuality (Connell and Dowsett 1992; Irvine 1995, 2–3).

Essentialism, as applied to human sexuality, firstly assumes that sexuality is a natural and inherent part of the individual. A common form of this belief is that individuals have a sexual drive or instinct which is presocial and which originates in human biology. There are at least three main reasons in support of such a belief. Firstly, it is compatible with Darwinian assumptions about the process of evolution and the biological need for species to reproduce and survive into the future (Levine 1984; Levine

1987; Laumann and Gagnon 1995, 185; Assiter 1996, 134). If such a sex drive did not exist, 'then there would be no biological imperative towards the survival of the species ...' (Assiter 1996, 134). This would violate Darwinian assumptions and require some other adequate form of explanation. Secondly, the sex drive appears to be similar, in some respects, to other biological needs such as for food and sleep. It is similar in that it appears and recurs in people independently of their intentions and actions. Some people report that this drive can be quite powerful or compelling even though there are various possibilities for ignoring, managing or gratifying it. Mohr (1992, 229) points out that it is unlikely the recurrence of the sex drive 'is the result of addiction or unconscious habit since many people have such drives who have never acted on them'. He suggests that the sex drive may be a non-intentional phenomenon 'that is modified, shaded, given various importance, but not overturned or voided by intentional acts' even though intentional acts are needed for sexual activity (Mohr 1992, 229). Thirdly, as a result of evolution, human beings have certain biological similarities with other species where mating behaviour *is* more evidently under biological imperatives. It is often assumed that, as a result of a common evolutionary history, humans might share some biological basis for sexual motivation with other species. On the other hand, however, biologists are also usually careful to point out the biological *differences* between humans and other species, and the greater role that learning and experience play in human decisions and actions involving sex (Pfaus 1999; Pfaus, Kippin and Coria-Avila 2003).

Over the last century, most sex researchers and theorists, including Havelock Ellis, Sigmund Freud, Alfred Kinsey, William Masters and Virginia Johnson have believed in the existence of an inherent sex drive. According to the psychiatrist, Richard von Krafft-Ebing (1921[1886], 1), for example, the 'propagation of the human species is not committed to accident or to the caprice of the individual, but made secure in a natural instinct, which, with all-conquering force and might, demands fulfillment.'

Sex researchers though, have often disagreed over whether the sex drive has biological and/or psychological origins and whether it is a product of genes, hormones or 'deep emotional influences' (Irvine 1995, 3). They also disagreed in their moral evaluation of the sex drive, such as whether it is a positive force distorted by an antagonistic society (for example, Ellis, Kinsey, Masters and Johnson) or a negative force which requires vigilant social control (for example, Freud and the majority of his followers). Nevertheless, the basic idea that sexuality is a powerful force within individuals was seldom questioned (Gagnon and Parker 1995, 7; Irvine 1995, 3).

The vast majority of the sexual theorists and researchers of this time also believed that there were fundamental differences between the sexuality of women and men which were grounded in their essentially different natures (Gagnon and Parker 1995, 7). This type of belief can still be found even in recent works:

Within the male the sex drive is more specific and direct. It tends to be isolated from feelings of love and affection and directed more towards orgasm. Within the female the sex drive is more diffuse and is related to feelings of affection. Indirect stimuli such as sexual fantasies and provocative pictures have a much greater effect on the male than the female. (cited in Irvine 1995, 4–5)

Essentialist views about human sexuality often include a second assumption that sexuality is 'predictably stable and similar both across cultures and throughout different historical times' (Irvine 1995, 11). This assumption is supposed to follow from the first assumption that sexuality is an inherent individual drive. This is because if sexuality is an innate individual drive, similar among human beings, or at least members of the same sex, then it will appear in much the same way largely irrespective of historical or social influences (Irvine 1995, 11). This second assumption is an example of a very strong form of essentialism which is sometimes known as 'biological reductionism' or 'biological determinism' (Irvine 1995, 3; Sayer 1997, 476).

PROBLEMS WITH ESSENTIALIST ACCOUNTS OF SEXUALITY

There are a number of serious deficiencies with essentialist perspectives on sexuality, including their accounts of sexual drives and instincts. Firstly, there is a problem with the claim that humans have a sexual drive which is rooted in their biology. There is so far no firm evidence that human desire for sexual activity is generated by a biological need. Researchers have tried to identify some kind of homeostatic disequilibrium in human bodily processes — such as in specific hormone levels or (in men) pressure on the seminal vesicles — to account for sexual need, however, no such disequilibrium has yet been conclusively identified (Person 1987, 395). According to Beach (1956, 4):

It used to be believed that prolonged sexual inactivity in adulthood resulted in the progressive accumulation of secretions within the accessory sex glands, and that nerve impulses from these distended receptacles gave rise to sexual urges. Modern evidence negates this hypothesis.

This means there is an important difference between people's need for sex and their need for food and water. In the latter case, it is possible to identify a disequilibrium in homeostatic bodily processes in which the biological need for food and water is experienced as hunger and thirst (Person 1987, 395). When an individual has been deprived of food, the body's stores of energy-producing substances, such as fats and sugars, 'are gradually depleted to maintain normal metabolism' (Beach 1956, 3). As food deprivation continues, the efficiency of the body's tissues are eventually impaired and a serious state of need develops. If food deprivation continues indefinitely, the result will be fatal. Water deprivation has analogous effects but they occur over a much shorter time period (Beach 1956, 3– 4). Beach (1956, 4) points out, however, that if an individual is deprived of a sexual outlet, he or she 'does not perish, regardless of the length of time involved.' Furthermore, it is not clear that the avoidance of sex *in itself* causes any illness, disability or tissue damage (Tiefer 1995, 13; Pfaus 1999, 125). The person who avoids sex misses out on 'a life experience that some people value very highly and most value at least somewhat' but avoiding sex does not seem to be ' "unhealthy" in the same way that avoiding protein is' (Tiefer 1995, 13). Conversely, participating in sexual activity does not necessarily preserve physical well-being (Pfaus 1999, 125).

There is also no evidence that an instinct governs human sexual *behaviour* (Zeitlin 1984, 43; Giddens 1989, 36; Laumann and Gagnon 1995, 186; Varela 2003). If the term 'instinct' refers to a genetically determined pattern of complex behaviour which appears in an animal at a particular point in its development, or in response to a particular environmental stimulus, then instincts only seem to exist in non-mammalian species (Laumann and Gagnon 1995, 185).

Sociological, anthropological and historical research has been particularly important in debunking instinct theories of human behaviour because it provided a wealth of counter-evidence to what people in Western societies believed was instinctive (Laumann and Gagnon 1995, 185). Sexual behaviour in humans seems to depend much more on experience and learning than on genetic or hormonal factors (Person 1987, 396). While it is true that certain neurophysiological organs and processes enable humans to engage in and experience sexual activities, humans have to learn *how* to engage in these activities (Zeitlin 1984, 44). As Ford and Beach (1952, 190) put it, 'the human male does not have to learn how to fill his penis with blood so that it becomes erect and rigid, but he may have to learn how to copulate....'

If a person has sexual feelings but has not learned what, if anything, to do about them, then there is nothing in human biology that will automatically lead him or her to have sexual intercourse. Zeitlin (1984, 44) underscores this point by referring to cases where individuals married each other without having any idea of how to have coitus. In one pertinent study, Dickinson and Beam (1970 [1931], 185– 6), for example, reported that eighteen of their one thousand patients remained virgins for an average of four years after marriage because, in almost all cases, neither the husband nor the wife knew how to have sexual intercourse.

The importance of the social context for learning about sexual expression is also highlighted by cases where humans have had little opportunity to learn about sexuality from other people. Zingg (1940), for example, reviewed thirty-one cases of humans who had lived in extreme isolation or with animals in the wild. Despite believing that human sexuality was closely linked to biology and a trait shared with other animals, Zingg (1940, 509) was surprised to find that, in socially isolated people, the sexual impulse was inhibited 'apparently due to unfamiliarity in the new situation [of human society] and impossibility in the old.' He concluded that:

> the social channeling of sex is much more necessary for its full expression than might be thought. Certainly this preponderating evidence of the inhibition of the sex impulse through isolation from social contact is surprizing, especially considering the other gross animal behavior of feral man in other urges, like hunger. (Zingg 1940, 510)

Given these problems with the notion of a sexual instinct, the concept of 'sexual drive' has sometimes been used to account for sexual behaviour. Sexual drive, in this sense, refers to 'behavior commonly exhibited by members of a species that appears to have a phylogenetic origin in the biological and neural evolution of the species' (Francoeur et al 1995, 168). This concept is sometimes preferred to that of sexual instinct because a drive is believed to be less deterministic than an instinct. The concept of drive, for example, is said to allow for variations in individual responses within a species (Francoeur et al 1995, 168– 9). Nevertheless, some drive theories are virtually indistinguishable from instinct theories of behaviour, and suffer from similar problems as the latter, namely, the lack of clear supporting evidence, the existence of counter examples to the theories, and the inability to specify the actual mechanisms by which a drive produces a particular form of behaviour (Laumann and Gagnon 1995, 186).

Other drive theories are more complex and have more of a bio-social character. Freud, for example, believed that 'libido' or sexual energy, is an unlearned or innate drive. During early childhood he thought its original sexual aim is inhibited and that it is culturally and psychically channelled toward different goals, such as love, work or artistic creation (Laumann and Gagnon 1995, 186). His attempt to distinguish between biological 'instincts' (primary or unlearned drives) and culturally and psychically shaped (secondary or learned) 'drives' had the potential to counter the bias of biological determinism in sexology. It also had the potential to facilitate a more sociological interpretation of sexual identity and behaviour. Ultimately, however, his theory of libido leaned more toward nature than culture, positing a fixed sexual drive which was largely independent of social structure (Kardiner, Karush and Ovesey 1966, 501–2; Stein 1989, 1).

The second problem with an essentialist view of sexuality is that it is unable to adequately explain what Freud called 'object choice' (Connell and Dowsett 1992, 54). Freud (1977a [1905], 45–6) defined the term 'sexual object' as 'the person from whom sexual attraction proceeds'. Instinct/

drive theories of sexuality might purport to explain why people want to have sex and the behaviour which results from this but they have little to say about variations in object choice even within the one society.

Thirdly, there is a problem with the strong essentialist claim that human sexuality is stable and similar for all people irrespective of historical or cultural context. While this view has little evidential support, if it was true, it would marginalise the impact of socio-cultural factors on human sexuality, and diminish the role of the social sciences in studying and explaining them. There is no reason, however, that essentialists have to make such an over-reaching claim, and, in fact, their claims are more defensible if they do not. As Sayer (1997, 478) points out:

> ... those who wish to argue that the body has certain essential properties, or at least causal powers, do not need to suppose that this entails a one-to-one relationship between a single biological essence and a single kind of behaviour ....

This is because, firstly, it is a mistake to think that biology only produces fixed and uniform behavioural outcomes. Perper (1985, 23) refers to this as a folklore version of biology which 'has nothing to do with' biology as a science. He points out that biology produces diversity, variability and change even in the behaviour of animals, such as rats, which were thought to have stereotypical mating interactions. Nor do genes 'program' behaviour. Rather, 'they create the *need* for one or more given behaviour patterns' (Perper 1985, 63; emphasis in original).

Secondly, biological essences, that is, biological capacities and powers, are subject to social and cultural mediation, as well as to human agency. As Sayer (1997, 478) explains:

> We have many biological powers, they can be activated and mediated in a vast number of ways, and hence the range of sexualities and other activities of which people are capable is wide, but like any social constructions behaviours draw partly on non-social materials, including the body, and are constrained and enabled by their properties.

This means that if sexuality is an inherent individual drive, then it does not follow that it will appear in all contexts in a similar way. It might not appear in a similar way, for example, if individuals have sex drives of different strengths, durations, and frequencies, if sex drives are affected by factors such as age, sex, illness, injury, stress or medication, or if the expression of sex drives is affected by experience, learning, opportunity or social approval. As Mohr (1992) points out, the existence of an inherent sex drive is quite compatible with diversity in the forms of its manifestation. Halwani (1998) has made a similar point in relation to an essentialist view of homosexual sexual orientation.

Furthermore, if the strong essentialist claim about sexual similarity and stability is accepted, then it might also mean that beliefs, attitudes and values about sexuality are falsely universalised from specific cultural groups in ways which are inaccurate and ethnocentric. This would assume without sufficient critical reflection that people in other times and places think and feel the same way that we might do about shared sexual practices (Irvine 1995, 11).

The fourth problem with essentialist accounts of human sexuality is that they have had little to say about pleasure and desire, topics which are common and important in representations of sexuality in art, music and literature (Connell and Dowsett 1992, 54–5; Pfaus 1999, 148). The notion of a sex drive or Freud's concept of libido is the closest essentialism comes to having a concept of desire. Pleasure has also been neglected as a feature of human experience being usually replaced by a 'discourse of nerve endings, engorged vesicles [and] muscular spasm' (Connell and Dowsett 1992, 55). The neglect of pleasure has been partially addressed by Abramson and Pinkerton's (1995) research which, among other things, considers its biological and psychological dimensions. However, an essentialist perspective on pleasure, grounded in biology or psychology, has to be adequate to its object of study, and this will probably mean that its account of pleasure is necessarily different to that of the arts or other disciplines.

Finally, an essentialist perspective on sexuality has been criticised for producing a 'degenerating' scientific research programme in the sense specified by Lakatos (1970). Lakatos (1970) argued that a research programme is a framework which guides future research in both a positive and negative way. 'The programme consists of methodological rules: some tell us what paths of research to avoid *(negative heuristic)*, and others what paths to pursue *(positive heuristic)*' (Lakatos 1970, 132). The negative heuristic of a programme contains the stipulation that its 'hard core' of basic assumptions must not be discarded or modified. This hard core of assumptions is protected from falsification by a 'protective belt' of auxiliary hypotheses. The positive heuristic, on the other hand, consists of various guidelines which suggest how the research programme might be developed. This involves supplementing the basic assumptions with additional assumptions in order to explain previously known facts and predict new phenomena. 'It is this protective belt... which has to bear the brunt of tests and get adjusted and re-adjusted, or even completely replaced, to defend the thus-hardened core' (Lakatos 1970, 133). A research programme can be regarded as progressive if it continues to predict novel facts and degenerating if it does not (Lakatos 1970).

Gagnon and Simon (1973, 7) argued as far back as the early 1970s that essentialist approaches to the study of sexuality were failing to provide new and cumulative research findings. Connell and Dowsett (1992, 54), too, argued that essentialism about sexuality has failed to provide an 'expanding program of investigation'. It is only able to continue by restricting itself to one small area of sexuality (the biological/physical dimension) which it regards as the most important but which is unable to account for phenomena in the remainder of the field (Connell and Dowsett 1992, 54). As Vance (1991, 879) puts it:

> The physiology of orgasm and penile erection no more explains a culture's sexual schema than the auditory range of the human ear explains its music. Biology and physical functioning are determinative only at the most extreme limits, and there to set the boundary of what is physically possible. The more interesting question for anthropological [and sociological] research on sexuality is to chart what is culturally possible - a far more expansive domain.

However, at least three points can be made in response to these criticisms. Firstly, essentialist approaches to sex research have not completely failed. Rather, they have had mixed success in their chosen areas. Pfaus (1999, 133–5), for example, points out that researchers now understand a great deal about endocrinology and reproductive physiology, that sexual behaviour in humans and other animals is influenced or governed by hormones and environmental factors, and that erection and ejaculation are similar physiological processes 'in many male mammals'. Furthermore, much of this progress has occurred in the last ten years (Pfaus et al 2003, 2). On the other hand, some things are poorly understood. Pfaus (1999, 134), for example, acknowledges that researchers understand very little about sexual desire, the role and evolution of female orgasm, or how orgasm might inhibit sexual desire or arousal.

Secondly, it is true that essentialist approaches to sexuality are typically associated with biological and psychological research programs, and that these programs are unlikely to account for the entire field of the 'sexual'. However, this is not a deficiency which is peculiar to essentialism. It is also true of non-essentialist approaches, and approaches grounded in other disciplines, such as the social sciences. The phenomena of sexuality contains biological, psychological and social dimensions, among others, and it is unrealistic to expect, for example, that a discipline concerned with the social can completely replace disciplines that are concerned with different objects of study (Mahoney 1983, ch. 2; Danermark 2001).

Thirdly, it is unclear to what extent the failures of essentialist research programmes on sexuality are due to failures of essentialism itself. Strong versions of essentialism involving, for example, biological reductionism or biological determinism are not defensible (Sayer 1997). However, some weaker versions of essentialism are at least as compatible with existing evidence as alternative accounts of sexuality (see, for example Mohr 1992; and Halwani 1998). On the other hand, there are clearly additional reasons for problems with essentialist research programmes, including 'scientific blinders', lack of cross-fertilisation between studies of human and animal

sexual behaviour, ethical and practical difficulties in experimentally studying human sexuality, and 'lack of sufficient technology' (Pfaus et al 2003,
2).

ESSENTIALISM, IDEOLOGY AND MEDICALISATION

Essentialism about sexuality may have had mixed results as a scientific
research programme but it remains a powerful ideology in society (Connell
and Dowsett 1992, 56). This ideology can take a myriad of different forms:
for example, that sexual orientation is the product of an inner sex drive;
that heterosexuality is natural and homosexuality unnatural; that men are
naturally sexually aggressive and women sexually passive; that male rape
of women or girls results from an uncontrollable male sex drive; that teen-
agers during puberty are 'driven' into sexual activity by their hormones
and so on (Irvine 1995, 4–7). In each of these cases biological 'grounds' are
used to support particular 'common-sense' beliefs about sexuality (Connell
and Dowsett 1992, 56).

'Medicalisation', a key aspect of medical social control, has been one of
the most important sources of support for essentialist views about sexuality. The term 'medicalisation' refers to three interrelated processes: firstly,
defining a particular issue as a health or medical problem; secondly, utilising
a biomedical theory to explain the 'problem'; and thirdly, using biomedical
measures or practices, such as drugs or surgery, to control or eliminate the
'problem'. The definitional process is arguably the most important since
without it the other two processes are unlikely to occur. Medicalisation,
however, can be regarded as occurring even if only the first process is evident. A wide variety of human experiences have been medicalised so that
they are now thought about in terms of health and disease. These include,
among others, childbirth, ageing, death, madness, illegal drug use, alcohol
drinking, eating problems, hyperactivity, learning difficulties, homosexuality, shoplifting and child abuse (Conrad 1992, 211–3; Conrad 2005). The
process has been so pervasive that Illich (1976) referred to it as the 'medicalisation of life'.

Sexuality has not been immune from the process of medicalisation. Over
the last century, the medical profession has increasingly come to dominate
discussions in this area. Previously, religious authorities and moral philosophers had been the experts, but by the late nineteenth century doctors
were redefining sexuality as a health issue (Weeks 1992, 221). They either
invented or helped disseminate new sexual categories, such as homosexuality and heterosexuality, which are now taken for granted by many people.
They also developed and promulgated a discourse of sexual disease containing concepts such as anorgasmia, impotence and sex addiction. These
days it is not uncommon for people to think of sexuality as a health issue,
particularly in the light of concern over the spread of sexually transmitted

diseases like Acquired Immune Deficiency Syndrome (AIDS) (Irvine 1995, 8).

Medicalisation encourages the tendency to regard sexuality as an internal drive by the way it positions sexuality as a health issue. In Western societies where the 'biomedical model' is dominant, health and illness are predominantly thought to be individual, biological experiences. The source of disease is often thought to be a specific aetiological agent, such as a bacterium, virus or parasite which invades the body and causes illness. Social, economic, political and environmental factors which might influence the distribution, onset, experience, management or outcome of ill health are frequently underestimated or ignored (Berliner 1985). When sexuality is medicalised, similar processes operate. For example, 'experts' who have defined too much sex as 'sex addiction' and too little sex as 'inhibited sexual desire disorder' may prefer to study human brains or hormones to find the causes of these 'diseases' rather than the social norms which influence people's ideas about what the proper or 'healthy' level of sexual activity should be. In these ways, the medicalisation of sexuality reinforces the idea that sexuality is just a natural and inherent property of the individual (Irvine 1995, 8–9).

SOCIAL CONSTRUCTIONISM

Social constructionism is the second major theoretical perspective for the study and interpretation of sexuality. It first emerged in the mid-1970s although it has earlier roots (Vance 1991, 878). The label itself can be traced back to Berger and Luckmann's (1966) famous treatise, *The Social Construction of Reality*. Generally, social constructionism has been less influential than essentialism which remains hegemonic in Western societies. Nevertheless, constructionism has gained a lot of acceptance among certain social groups including sociologists, historians, anthropologists, feminists, and lesbian and gay scholars and activists (Vance 1989; Vance 1991; Brickell 2006).

Social constructionism has many and diverse intellectual roots which cannot be exhaustively charted here. Philosophically, however, certain key constructionist ideas can be traced back to the work of the German scholar, Immanuel Kant (1724–1804). Two of Kant's ideas, in particular, are important: 'the idea of an unknowable, noumenal world independent of us; and the idea of the known phenomenal world as partly our creation through the imposition of concepts' (Devitt 1991, 235). The third key constructionist idea — relativism — was foreign to Kant. Relativism is the view that there are many different traditions and forms of human life, each of which produces its own standards, for example, of truth, goodness and beauty. Relativists typically believe that none of these traditions or ways of life can be understood or judged by criteria which belongs to a different tradition (Trigg 1985, 17). When the three ideas referred to above are combined, social constructionism can be defined as a perspective which rests on the following central beliefs:

> The only independent reality is beyond the reach of our knowledge and language. A known world is partly constructed by the imposition of concepts. These concepts differ from (linguistic, social, scientific, etc) group to group, and hence the worlds of groups differ. Each such world exists only relative to an imposition of concepts. (Devitt 1991, 235)

Social constructionism has also developed from or been influenced in various ways by a number of other intellectual traditions and theoretical approaches. These include, among others, symbolic interactionism, labelling theory, symbolic anthropology, existential and phenomenological sociology, dramaturgical sociology, the sociology of knowledge, ethnomethodology, pragmatism, literary deconstruction and various social psychological theories (Gergen 1985; Gagnon and Parker 1995, 8; Heartfield 1996; Brickell 2006). From these many and varied sources a more general theoretical framework known as social constructionism gradually emerged.

Gergen (1985) has identified four main metatheoretical assumptions which most social constructionist work is based on. Firstly, people's experiences of the world do not in themselves determine how the world will be understood. This assumption stems from the critique of positivist-empiricist views of knowledge in which scientific theory is seen as a direct reflection of reality. Social constructionism encourages scepticism towards the idea that taken for granted categories and understandings are simply derived from observation and it attempts to challenge the idea that accepted knowledge is objective. For example, Kessler and McKenna's (1978) work challenges the supposed fact that there are only two genders. By examining variations in the way different social groups understand gender their work opens up new possibilities for rethinking gender differences or of completely abandoning gender distinctions (Gergen 1985, 266–7).

Secondly, the concepts and categories which people use to understand the world differ quite considerably over time and between cultures. Concepts such as the child, romantic love, knowledge, self and identity, for example, have had different meanings attached to them by people in different times and places. This is of particular interest to social constructionists who want to study the historical and cultural bases of various constructions of reality (Gergen 1985, 267–8).

Thirdly, the extent to which particular beliefs persist over time or remain popular has less to do with their level of empirical support and more to do with their usefulness to particular individuals or social groups. Such usefulness can occur in any number of ways including the assistance of rhetoric, negotiation, conflict, political influence or social control (Gergen 1985,

268). Tiefer (1987, 72) provides a telling example of the way in which a 'positivist-empiricist model of psychological research has been criticised for its limitations and omissions, yet ... persists because of prestige, tradition and unexamined congruence with cultural values'.

Fourthly, descriptions and explanations of the world are themselves forms of social action and they produce social effects (Gergen 1985, 268). To 'construct' certain people as sexually or racially inferior to others, for example, is to encourage certain social responses toward them and not others. Similarly, to describe someone as a 'malingerer', for example, has very different social implications from describing her or him as genuinely ill, particularly if the description is provided by a doctor within the context of a worker's compensation claim.

In summary, then, social constructionists generally believe that meaning is not a fixed and inherent part of the world and that people's experiences of the world do not by themselves determine how they will understand the world. People understand their experiences through socially created concepts and meanings (or 'frames'). Different social groups have different concepts and meanings for understanding their experiences and with them they construct different versions of reality. What counts as knowledge or as reality in one society, may not be accepted as such in another. Social constructionist researchers typically want to investigate how and why certain meanings (and not other meanings) are attached to people's experiences, how and why meanings change, and (for some constructionists) how meanings might assist or hinder some social groups in dominating other social groups (Gergen 1985; Conrad and Schneider 1985).

SOCIAL CONSTRUCTIONISM AND SEXUALITY

> Social construction theory in the field of sexuality proposed an extremely outrageous idea. It suggested that one of the last remaining outposts of the 'natural' in our thinking was fluid and changeable, the product of human action and history rather than the invariant result of the body, biology or an innate sex drive. (Vance 1989, 13)

The development of social construction theory over the last thirty or so years has provided a new theoretical perspective with which to challenge the hegemony of essentialist views of sexuality. The basic idea of social construction theory as applied to sexuality is that sexuality is a product or construct of various social and cultural influences operating within particular historical contexts (Irvine 1995, 12). Social constructionists might differ as to what might be constructed, for example, sexual desire, object choice, sexual acts, identities or communities but they share the desire to question and problematise sexuality as a field of inquiry (Vance 1991, 878).

While essentialists tend to view sexuality as a fixed essence which does not alter over time or through different cultural contexts, social constructionists would reject any universal definitions of sexuality. They would argue instead that what people regard as sexual and what sexuality means can vary greatly over time or from place to place (Irvine 1995, 12–13). The basic constructionist position is that 'nothing is sexual but naming makes it so. Sexuality is a social construct learnt in interaction with others' (Plummer 1975, 30). Plummer (1975, 30–1) illustrates this point with two very different scenarios: a man fingering the vagina of a woman who is lying naked; and a boy who is watching a game of football. Plummer suggests that if one was asked to say which situation was sexual, then the first situation would intuitively seem to be sexual while the second one would not. Yet if one focused on the actors' definitions of the situation rather than their overt behaviour then a very different answer might emerge. The man fingering the woman's genitals might be a doctor carrying out a gynaecological examination, and the doctor and the woman might have clearly defined their interaction in medical terms. On the other hand, the boy watching the game of football might feel sexual desire for the football players and be fantasising about the players engaging in various sexual acts with him. Plummer (1975, 31) goes on to ask:

> When a child plays with its genitals, is this 'sexual'? When a person excretes is this sexual? When a man kisses another man publicly is this sexual? When a couple are naked together, is this sexual?... When a man and woman copulate out of curiosity or out of duty, is this sexual?... Most of the situations above could be defined as sexual by members; [but] they need not be.

The problematic nature of sexual meanings and the way they are assigned is one of the key reasons why social constructionists are interested in studying how and why different beliefs, attitudes and practices come to be labelled and understood as sexual in different times and places. It is also why social constructionists are more interested in understanding the social and cultural aspects of sexuality rather than in studying the individual who is abstracted from his/her social context and which essentialists tend to regard as the most important element in explaining sexuality. To the extent that constructionists are interested in the sexuality of individuals it is with individuals in particular socio-historical settings (Irvine 1995, 12–13).

A second key area of disagreement between essentialists and constructionists is over the notion of a sex instinct or drive. While essentialists usually posit the existence of a pre-social sex instinct or drive, most constructionists downplay or even question the existence of this supposedly innate force. The most radical constructionists would deny there is any inherent sexual instinct or drive and instead would see sexual desire itself as historically and culturally constructed from the capacities and energies of the body. If this position is taken, then important questions still remain about how this actually happens. More moderate constructionists, on the other hand, might accept some notion of inherent desire but see it as socially constructed in terms of actions, identity, object choice and/or community (Vance 1991, 878).

A related area of contention is that of object choice, or the direction of sexual interest, for example, whether heterosexual, homosexual or bisexual. The more radical constructionists would deny that the direction of erotic interest is intrinsic to or inherent in the individual and would argue that it is constructed from the individual's polymorphous capabilities. Other constructionists, however, would hold that the direction of sexual interest is fixed but that the behavioural form of this interest might vary because it is influenced by cultural context, subjective experience or opportunities for sexual expression (Vance 1991, 878).

The debate over sexuality between essentialists and constructionists is sometimes misconstrued as just another form of the nature-nurture debate (Irvine 1995, 15). In this latter debate there are two extreme positions: geneticism which is the view that individual or group characteristics can be entirely explained in terms of genetic inheritance; and cultural determinism, the position that such characteristics can be exclusively explained in terms of culture and socialisation (Abercrombie et al 1994, 279). Most researchers today would agree that these two extreme views are untenable and that human behaviour is influenced by a complex interaction of cultural and biological factors. Disagreements tend to centre on the extent, and the ways in which biological or cultural factors influence behaviour (Vance 1991, 883).

Proponents of the view that the essentialist-constructionist debate is simply another version of the nature-nurture debate suggest that sexual essentialism is similar to the argument from nature (e.g. geneticism), while social constructionism is similar to the argument from nurture (e.g. cultural determinism). However, while there may be similarities between the essentialist and nature positions, it is a mistake to fully equate social construction theory with the nurture side of the debate in which sexual desires and object choice are held to be learned rather than inborn. The reason for this is that social construction theory goes beyond (although it includes) an argument for cultural causation. Social construction theory also insists on deconstructing and critically examining the very condition or behaviour which both the nature and nurture proponents have usually taken for granted as unproblematic and which they are trying in different ways to explain. That is, social constructionists typically insist that the object of study itself requires just as much critical analysis as any supposed causal mechanisms that may have produced it (Vance 1991, 883; Irvine 1994, 244).

SOME MISGUIDED CRITICISMS OF
SOCIAL CONSTRUCTIONISM

Vance (1989, 15–18) has outlined a number of unhelpful criticisms of social construction theory which are generally based on misunderstandings of this perspective. These criticisms must be examined and answered if such misconceptions are to be avoided and more fruitful evaluation of construction theory is to occur.

Firstly, social construction theory is sometimes criticised for allegedly suggesting that sexual identity, particularly lesbian and gay identity, is somehow not as important or real if it is socially constructed as opposed to being biologically determined. This criticism misses the point that it is possible to explain how people's understanding of reality is at least partly socially constructed without implying that these understandings are not real or important for the people who rely on them. Nevertheless, it is true to say that when people understand social construction theory they have at least the potential to question taken for granted naturalistic beliefs about sexuality including, perhaps, their own essentialist conceptions of identity (Vance 1989, 16).

Secondly, critics sometimes contend that, according to social construction theory, individual sexual identity is under conscious control, that it can easily be changed like changing a set of clothes, and that the large scale social organisation of sexuality can also be easily altered. Social constructionists, however, generally do not subscribe to these views. There is usually no suggestion that individuals who are socialised within one cultural tradition can simply shed their culture and take on another at whim. Social constructionists would not deny that individuals may experience changes and fluidity in their sexuality but their work does not necessarily imply that individuals have an open ended ability to reconstruct their sexuality over a lifetime. Nor do social constructionists generally suggest that large scale institutional features of sexuality in society can be quickly or easily changed just because sexuality is socially constructed (Vance 1989, 16–17).

Finally, some critics have exaggerated the social constructionist preoccupation with change and differences in beliefs, attitudes and practices to suggest that social constructionism is opposed to recognising or acknowledging stability and similarities in meanings and behaviour. However, the constructionist interest in change and difference does not require such a researcher to always find it nor does it prevent the discovery of continuities and similarities (Vance 1989, 17).

PROBLEMS WITH SOCIAL CONSTRUCTION THEORY

There are a number of important problems with social construction theory both in relation to its philosophical underpinnings and in its specific application to the field of sexuality. In the latter case, three main problems have been identified.

Firstly, the increasing popularity and widespread use of the term 'social constructionism' may make it seem that social constructionism is a unified and unique theoretical perspective which all self-identified social constructionists share. The problem is that the use of this term can help to obscure the differences between various social constructionist writers. All of them may reject transcultural and transhistorical definitions of sexuality and hold that sexuality is influenced by historical and cultural factors but there are many differences (as noted above) as to what social constructionist writers might believe is socially constructed. This might include such phenomena as sexual desire, object choice, identity, acts, communities and even sexuality itself. The differences between social constructionist writers means that it is important to discriminate between them as to what each one believes is socially constructed and also to be clear about how the term is used in one's own work (Vance 1989, 18–21; Brickell 2006).

Secondly, if sexuality is purely a social construction and can have multiple meanings in multiple discourses then what, if anything, gives these discourses a common point of reference which would allow the term to be used comparatively in a meaningful way (Vance 1989, 21; Mohr 1992, 236)? As Vance (1989, 21) puts it, the object of study itself 'becomes evanescent and threatens to disappear'. Some social constructionists, such as Michel Foucault have tried to totally deconstruct sexuality as a category and have run into this very problem (Morrow 1995). Others have sought to avoid it by assuming that certain types of behaviour and physical interactions can be reliably regarded as sexual even though they are found in different cultures and historical periods (Vance 1989, 21–3).

The third problem concerns the role of the body in social construction theory. Social construction theory has been very useful in challenging the dominance of essentialist views that sexuality is simply a natural part of being human and is a product of biology. Yet as certain forms of social construction theory stress that sexual desire and impulse are culturally created there seems to be less and less room in such theory for bodily anatomy and physiology. What is the role of biology in people's sexual lives and how can the body be properly conceptualised within social construction theory without lapsing back into biological determinist forms of essentialism (Vance 1989, 23)?

Those with essentialist views of sexuality tend to study the body because they believe it is the locus of truth about sexuality. Social constructionists, on the other hand, tend to regard the body as providing the physical basis of and potential for engaging in and experiencing various sexual acts. In their view, the body not only provides energy for sexual practices but is itself a site for the enactment and experience of various thoughts, feelings and behaviours which are regarded as sexual within a particular culture (Irvine 1995, 16). The body can also impose limits on a person's sexual expression. For example, if a male does not develop an erection, or if a female does not have a penetrable vagina, then there are limits as to what sexual activities they can engage in. At the same time, however, it is important not to over-estimate the biological dimension of sexuality (Mahoney 1983, 24). This is because it is people's culture which teaches them how to utilise the body's potential in order to 'construct' themselves as sexual beings (Irvine 1995, 16).

Social constructionists sometimes compare sexuality to music as a way of illustrating both the interplay between biology and culture, and the often unique way that sexuality is treated within society. A properly functioning ear and sensory system are needed for hearing but the music which can be heard and enjoyed is a product of culture. In this case, people do not usually think that their experience of music can be explained solely in terms of ear structure and function, that a preference for classical music over heavy metal can be found somewhere in the brain, or that an indifference to certain types of music means there is a physical dysfunction with the ears. Yet in the case of sexuality, its truth has been predominantly sought in the body, sexual preference has been sought in the brain, and indifference to certain forms of sexual activity has been treated as having a physical basis. Social constructionists would tend to hold that the essentialist desire to find the truth of sexuality in the body is itself likely to be a culturally constructed belief (Irvine 1995, 16, 18).

Nevertheless, Irvine (1995, 17–18) goes on to suggest that there are a number of ways in which the body can be regarded as a 'social construct'. Firstly, the body does not remain totally static and immune from social influences over time. Stress, for example, can alter body chemistry, and severe emotional traumas can physically affect the makeup of the brain (Irvine 1995, 17). This suggests that biological and social processes do not simply converge at a 'boundary between the body and society' but that internal bodily processes can already be, in part, social products (Connell and Dowsett 1992, 73).

Secondly, people's experiences of their own embodiment are greatly influenced by the societies in which they live. Most cultures contain beliefs about beauty, for example, which can make some people feel proud of and happy with their bodies and others feel ashamed or uncomfortable. People who deviate from culture-bound ideals of beauty, such as very tall or short people, very fat or thin people, people with disabilities or the very old may feel that life can be a socially difficult or unpleasant experience (Irvine 1995, 17–18).

Finally, scientific ideas about the anatomy and physiology of the body have not always been based on objective knowledge. Social, economic and political influences have shaped the processes and outcomes of scientific research so that, for example, science has often wrongly produced sexist and racist research findings which have served to bolster and legitimise pre-existing social inequalities (Irvine 1995, 18; Heartfield 1996, 10–11).

Yet while Irvine (1995, 17–18) makes some useful points about the way in which social factors can affect the understanding, experience and workings of the body, there is something very misleading about the way she (and other social constructionist writers) refer to the body as a social construct. The body, of course, is not literally constructed out of social phenomena, such as discourses, norms or cultural practices. What social construction theory generally needs is an explicitly realist conception of the body as something which exists independently of the various discourses about it and which is not reducible to them. The body is a product of nature and a material entity which is also experienced subjectively. It has its own structures, processes and causal powers which provide the necessary conditions for human experience and practice, including sexuality. These properties and powers are themselves part of the object of the biological and natural sciences (Soper 1995, 132–3, 135).

At the same time, however, as social constructionist writers emphasise, the body is usually experienced and lived within a social context. It is experienced, at least in part, through the mediation of culturally constructed discourses, and is materially shaped and moulded by specific cultural practices (Soper 1995, 137). One of the strengths of social constructionism is in the way it draws our attention to, and helps us to understand, these processes. However, there is no reason it cannot perform these tasks effectively without lapsing into conceptions of the body which occlude its physical reality or which render it as ontologically dependent on or reducible to the effects of discourse.

Having now examined some of the key theoretical problems which arise from the way that social construction theory has been applied to the substantive area of sexuality, it is now necessary to discuss a different though related set of problems with the theory which concern the basic philosophical assumptions on which it rests. There are a number of problems to consider.

The first problem is that the Kantian notion of noumenal things-in-themselves is useless as a basis for explanation and is also incoherent. Constructionists like to refer to things-in-themselves because they seem to provide an external constraint on theorising. While it seems plausible to believe that there is such an external constraint, the notion of things-in-themselves does not seem to provide it. If we cannot know anything about things-in-themselves, as constructionists typically maintain, then we cannot know anything about how they exercise constraint. Nor can we predict or explain such constraint. In terms of Kant's own views, the very notion of the noumenal world exercising causal constraint on human theorising is itself incoherent because he believed that causality is a concept imposed on the world by human beings. That is, it is part of the phenomenal world rather than the noumenal world (Devitt 1991, 237–8).

There is a modified version of constructionism which holds that it is not possible to provide an account of the constraints on theorising. This can take the form of the implausible view that there are no constraints on theorising and that we can think whatever we like regardless of how the world actually is, or the view that there are constraints but that in principle we cannot say anything about them. The latter position only avoids incoherence at the cost of silence (Devitt 1991, 238).

A second and more serious problem concerns the constructionist idea that we make the known world of sticks and stones, cats, trees and mountains with our concepts. As Devitt (1991, 238) puts it:

> How could cookie cutters in the head literally carve out cookies in dough that is outside the head? How could dinosaurs and stars be dependent on the activities of our minds? It would be crazy to claim that there were no dinosaurs or stars before there were people to think about them. Constructionists do not seem to claim this. But it is hardly any less crazy to claim that there *would not have been* dinosaurs or stars if there *had not been* people (or similar thinkers). And this claim seems essential to Constructivism: unless it were so, dinosaurs and stars could not be dependent on us and our minds. (emphasis in original)

Thirdly, there is the problem of relativism. Relativists deny that it is possible to conceive of any kind of independent reality. Reality, for them, is whatever people believe it is, and since different people hold different conceptions of reality relativists think there must, in fact, be different realities. The fundamental problem with relativism is that it is self-referentially incoherent. This is because it presents its own claims as being universally true rather than being relatively true, for example, by asserting as objectively true that all truth is relative. That is, if relativists maintain that it is impossible to have objective knowledge of a reality which is independent of the knower then it seems they cannot avoid falling into inconsistency by assuming that their relativist thesis itself is a form of objective knowledge (Trigg 1973, 2–3; Flew 1984, 303; Pojman 1995, 690).

Devitt (1991, 237) has argued that the claims of constructionism seem so '*prima facie* absurd as to prompt a search for a non-literal, charitable way of interpreting them' (emphasis in original). He suggests that a metaphorical interpretation of certain claims might be more suitable. For instance, he suggests that when constructionists talk about the social construction of reality or of the world they are really referring to the construction of *theories* about the world. There is little doubt, that theories and concepts can be regarded as human constructions. Similarly, when constructionists talk of imposing theories on the world they are really referring to the way the mind imposes theories on our *experiences* of the world. And when constructionists claim that X exists relative to a particular theory they are actually claiming that there is a *concept* of X within the theory (Devitt 1991, 239).

Charitable interpretations of social construction theory seem to be required because of the careless way in which many constructionists confuse talk about theories with talk about the world. Kuhn (1970, 115), for example, seems to be saying that when astronomers changed their minds about how to interpret the discovery of Uranus — first regarding it as a star, then a comet, and finally a planet — that the universe itself changed and that 'there were [now] several fewer stars and one more planet in the world of the professional astronomer'. Since it is absurd to think that a consensus among astronomers could actually destroy stars and create a planet it seems best not to interpret Kuhn's statements literally (Devitt 1991, 239).

Being charitable to social constructionists, however, can have its own problems. In the first place, some constructionists are aware of the distinction between talk about theories and talk about the world yet they often continue to claim that when things look different as a result of theory change that they are really different as well. Secondly, the famous constructionist thesis of the incommensurability of paradigms would no longer be viable if constructionism was interpreted charitably. This is because if competing theories do not create their own worlds but are merely accounts of the one world then the theories could actually be compared. Finally, some constructionists leave no option for interpreting their work charitably because they so openly and explicitly defend what seem to be absurd positions (Devitt 1991, 240–1). An example of such a position is that of Nelson Goodman (1980, 213) who says:

> we do not make stars as we make bricks; not all making is a matter of moulding mud. The worldmaking mainly in question here is making not with hands but with minds, or rather with languages or other symbol systems. *Yet when I say that worlds are made, I mean it literally....* (emphasis added)

These problems with social constructionism underline the fact that there is an important difference between those who believe that people 'construct' reality out of their theories, concepts, language or experience, and those who start from the position that whatever exists does so whether or not people are able to conceive of it (Trigg 1980, vii). Constructionists typically blur the distinction between reality and what people believe about it. They confuse talk about theories of the world with talk about the world itself. Constructionist discourse, however, can only be regarded as true if it is metaphorically about theories rather than the world but this would mean that its distinctive theses, such as the incommensurability of paradigms can no longer be sustained (Devitt 1991, 241).

It is scepticism about the accessibility of reality, as suggested by the constructionist reliance on the unknowable Kantian noumena (things-in-themselves), which leads constructionists away from questions about the relationship between truth and reality to a focus on what people believe to be true. When human beliefs vary so markedly over time and from place to place it is easy to believe that this is because of the different social backgrounds of the people holding these beliefs. Such differences will then need to be explained by a relevant social science discipline, such as sociology or anthropology. The problem for the sociologist who operates from a social constructionist position which denies access to objective reality is how to avoid the self-contradiction of then assuming that his or her own causal explanations (about the impact of social influences on individual belief) are objectively true. If such a sociologist is to be consistent, she or he must recognise that sociological explanations are as much the product of social conditioning as any other type of belief or explanation, and that they are equally susceptible to further sociological study. The problem that then arises is that of an infinite regress. A sociologist will never be able to make a claim to truth if such social constructionist assumptions are justified. Any claims made will only be what the sociologist believes and these can simply be shown by another sociologist to be socially conditioned (Trigg 1989, 124–5; Mohr 1992, 242; Craib 1997, 10).

Social constructionists, then, seem to be caught in a dilemma. If they adhere to the view that sociologists can never know reality and can only deal with beliefs which are socially conditioned then they must also apply this to themselves. This will make their work of little significance to other people because there would be 'no compelling reason why they should accept what are merely the socially conditioned prejudices of others' (Trigg 1989, 132). Alternatively, a social constructionist may concede that access to reality is possible and that people can partially escape cultural prejudice and social pressure. In this case, the constructionist can consistently claim that his or her research findings are true but there is a cost. His or her subject area will be more limited 'since social pressure or any other kind of causation, is not wholly explanatory if rational consideration of evidence is possible' (Trigg 1989, 132).

In light of the serious problems with the strong form of social constructionism which have just been outlined, my argument must of necessity rely on a heavily modified form of constructionism which is closer to the latter position described by Trigg (1989) above. This modified form of social constructionism has no need to deny that epistemological access to reality is possible and so it avoids the problems associated with a useless and incoherent Kantian notion of things-in-themselves as well as the problem of relativism. It also insists on maintaining the distinction between reality and how people conceive of it in order to escape the absurdity of those constructionist claims which confuse the two and end up stating, for example, that theories somehow literally create their own worlds. There is nothing wrong in principle, however, with the social constructionist project of trying to understand the way in which social influences affect the construction of scientific theories or the way that culture affects how people interpret their experiences of the world. This has already been conceded in the discussion of how constructionist claims can be regarded as true if they are considered in a metaphorical rather than a literal sense. Furthermore, social constructionism need not be used for the extreme purpose of trying to show that all scientific or other knowledge claims are merely fictions constructed from social conventions. Its value in guiding research is in the way it helps to challenge common-sense and positivist notions of science in which science is held to be infallible or the only path to truth (Azevedo 1997). Social construction theory does not predict what particular answers will be found during research but it is committed to asking new questions 'and to challenging assumptions which impair our ability to even imagine these questions' (Vance 1989, 15).

CONCLUSION

This chapter has reviewed and evaluated two of the major theoretical perspectives on human sexuality: essentialism and social constructionism. Essentialism has its origins in ancient philosophical thought but has been applied in certain ways to the study and analysis of human sexuality. It generally assumes that sexuality is a natural and inherent part of the individual (commonly expressed in the notion that individuals have a biologically based sexual drive or instinct), and that sexuality is fairly stable and similar (perhaps allowing for gender differences) among people in different times and places. It is the dominant, though not unchallenged, way of thinking about sexuality in Western societies.

This chapter has criticised the essentialist approach to sexuality in a number of areas: in terms of its account of sexual instincts and drives, its inability to adequately account for sexual object choice, pleasure and desire, and the inability of strong versions of essentialism to explain diversity and change in human sexuality. Essentialism has had mixed results in its scientific research programmes but it remains powerful as an ideology within society. This ideology is buttressed by processes, such as the medicalisation of human experiences and problems.

Social constructionism was the other major theoretical perspective discussed in this chapter. It first emerged in the mid-1970s but has earlier roots in disciplines such as philosophy, sociology, anthropology and psychology. It has gained considerable acceptance among certain social groups, such as sociologists, anthropologists and historians, and has often been presented as a critique of, and alternative to, essentialism. Social constructionists generally stress the way in which meanings and learning about sexuality are shaped by the sociocultural context although constructionist writers often differ over what, and how far, various phenomena are 'constructed'.

This chapter has discussed some of the generally misguided criticisms of social constructionism, such as its alleged suggestion that socially constructed sexual identities are not as real as biologically determined ones;

that sexual identity and social structural aspects of sexuality can be easily altered; and that social construction theory is unable to cope with stability and similarity in sexual meanings and behaviour. However, there are more substantial criticisms which relate both to its philosophical underpinnings and its application to human sexuality. In the latter case, it has been argued that the increasing use of the term 'social constructionism' tends to obscure important differences among constructionist writers; that the more sexuality is regarded as having been socially constructed the more it threatens to disappear as an object of study; and that the more the body is regarded as a social construct the more its material reality is occluded or is reduced to an effect of discourse or cultural practices. In the case of social constructionism's philosophical underpinnings, the main problems concern its assumptions that reality is unknowable, that humans make the known world with their concepts, and that truth is a relative rather than objective phenomenon.

This chapter has argued that if social constructionism is going to be defensible and useful as a theoretical perspective then it needs to be explicitly grounded in realist philosophical assumptions that reality exists independently of human conceptions of it, and that, in principle, it is accessible to human knowledge. Once social constructionism is grounded in these assumptions, it will avoid unnecessary aporias, without losing its value in guiding the critical analysis of 'scientific' work, such as that of Masters and Johnson. The following chapter initiates the discussion of their work in relation to their laboratory research on human sexual physiology.

4 Masters and Johnson's Research on Human Sexual Response

INTRODUCTION

The concept of sexual functioning is central to the theory and practice of sex therapy. This concept refers to a standard of sexual health from which sexual dysfunctions can be distinguished. William Masters and Virginia Johnson are generally acknowledged to be the most important researchers to have provided scientific evidence on human sexual functioning. They revolutionised sex research in the second half of the twentieth century by directly studying the sexual responses of 694 research volunteers under laboratory conditions. The report of this research, *Human Sexual Response* (1966), was hailed as ground breaking and its publication caused reverberations around the world.

The aim of this chapter is to provide a review of the rationale, conduct, major findings and public impact of Masters and Johnson's (1966) research. The chapter begins by examining their research rationale. It is argued that the research rationale was explicitly designed to facilitate the development of sex therapy and to address pressing public concerns about divorce and the break down of the family unit in U.S. society. The chapter then describes the funding, location and main research questions of the 'Sex Research Project'. It is argued that Masters and Johnson's research approach was modelled on that of scientific medicine and that this approach was useful both in furthering their objectives and in gaining legitimacy for their project. Following this, the chapter discusses the significance of the initial research with prostitutes and the main reasons for the unrepresentative sample of volunteers who were studied in the main phase of this research. The chapter then outlines the nature, duration and major findings of the research. The chapter concludes by arguing that Masters and Johnson's research received a very positive public reception and that, where criticism occurred, it focused more on their methods of investigation than their actual research findings. It is argued that the findings themselves were generally accepted as fact by a number of different audiences for a number of different reasons.

RESEARCH RATIONALE

William Masters (1915–2001) was a U.S. medical specialist trained in obstetrics and gynaecology. Prior to his work on human sexual response, he carried out research on a variety of topics, including the oestrous cycle of the female rabbit and hormone replacement therapy for postmenopausal women (Brecher and Brecher 1967, 41–3). His study of the anatomy and physiology of human sexual response began in 1954. It was located in Washington University's Department of Obstetrics and Gynecology in the School of Medicine (Masters and Johnson 1966, 3). This study was originally known as the 'Sex Research Project' and later as the 'Reproductive Biology Research Project' (Brecher and Brecher 1967, 43).

There were three main reasons for the Sex Research Project. Firstly, Masters argued that there was little scientific information about human sexual response. Prevailing social mores meant it was easier for researchers to study sexual response in non-human animals. However, Masters was dissatisfied with the relevance of these studies to humans. He proposed to overcome this problem by directly studying human sexual response in the laboratory. He wanted to accumulate definitive scientific information on sexual functioning and to debunk existing fallacies on the topic (Masters and Johnson 1966; Masters et al 1985, 20).

Contrary to popular belief, Masters and Johnson were not the first researchers to directly study human sexual response. There were many others before them. They included F. Roubaud (France); G. Klumbies, H. Kleinsorge and A. Wernich (Germany); H. Mitsuya et al (Japan); T. H. Van de Velde (The Netherlands); R. G. Bartlett Jr., J. Beck, E. P. Boas, R. L. Dickinson, E. F. Goldschmidt, E. Grafenberg, A. C. Kinsey, A. Mosovich, P. F. Munde, B. S. Talmey and J. B. Watson (United States) (Brecher 1970, 287–94; Rowland 1999, 3). The impression that human sexual response had not been previously studied was probably due to the fact that earlier sex researchers tended to keep their work secret. This was to minimise the potential of negative public reaction, ostracism by peers and disruption to research projects and careers (Irvine 1990b, 11–12).

By the middle of the twentieth century, there was actually a great deal of research on heart rates during coitus, the effect of orgasm on blood pressure, reproduction and metabolic rates, and even electroencephalograms of brain-wave activity during sexual arousal and orgasm (Brecher 1970, 287–94). Unfortunately, however, this body of research was flawed in a number of ways. It was often based on tiny, even atypical, samples. It focused only on selected aspects of sexual response. Recording instruments were rarely used. There were unsystematic and even conflicting eye witness accounts of physiological processes. Researchers also sometimes relied on anecdotal information. Masters' aim in his research was to raise the study of 'sexual physiology to a level of reliability comparable to that long since achieved by cardiac and gastrointestinal physiology' (Brecher 1970, 294).

The second reason for the Sex Research Project was that Masters wanted to use his scientific information on normal human sexual response as a baseline for understanding and treating human sexual inadequacy.

> When the laboratory program for the investigation of human sexual functioning was designed in 1954, permission to constitute the program was granted upon a research premise which stated categorically that the greatest handicap to successful treatment of sexual inadequacy was a lack of reliable physiological information in the area of human sexual response. (Masters and Johnson 1970, 1)

Masters and Johnson (1966) attempted to justify their laboratory research by arguing that sexual inadequacy had caused a crisis in U.S. society by undermining marriage and the family. They echoed the view that sexual inadequacy within the marital unit was the 'greatest single cause of family unit destruction and divorce', and maintained that the problem was so extensive it was beyond the capacity of the relevant 'helping' professions to deal with (Masters and Johnson 1966, vi). They admitted, however, that they had no accurate epidemiological evidence on the incidence of sexual dysfunction in the United States. However, they said 'a conservative estimate would indicate half the marriages as either presently sexually dysfunctional or imminently so in the future' (Masters and Johnson 1970, 369). They presented themselves as the potential saviours of U.S. society through their scientific approach to sexual inadequacy. This approach, they hoped, would eliminate sexual dysfunction within the following decade and render their book on the topic obsolete in the process (Masters and Johnson 1970, v).

It is not too difficult to see one of the key reasons why Masters and Johnson harnessed their research on sexual physiology to saving social institutions, such as marriage and the family. Sex research for most of its history has been a somewhat disreputable endeavour. As a consequence, researchers wanting to study in this area have had to find ways to circumvent or minimise opposition which might halt or otherwise interfere with their work. One strategy often adopted by sex researchers has been to investigate important medical or social problems which have a sexual component to them. Usually this has not been too difficult because many kinds of sexual behaviours themselves have often been regarded as medical or social problems (Mahoney 1983, 34). By promising to use their scientific research to save the institutions of marriage and the family, and to help preserve the existing social order, Masters and Johnson could simultaneously further their own objectives. They could ease the passage of their research, increase their chances of attracting and maintaining research funding, enhance the legitimacy and profile of sexology, and generate support from social groups also concerned with the same social 'problems', such as divorce and family breakdown.

Masters and Johnson aimed to use their research on sexual physiology to tackle human sexual inadequacy in two main ways. The first way was through better sex education. They hoped that once they had discovered the truth about human sexual response, their findings could be disseminated to the public via clinicians and the media. This information could then be used by people to improve their sex lives and marriages. Masters, for example, worked as a consultant for *Playboy* magazine's Adviser (Heidenry 1997, 284), and he and Johnson also conducted symposia with married couples, in the early 1970s, in order to prevent the occurrence of sexual dysfunctions. Some of these symposia later formed the basis of their book, *The Pleasure Bond* (1980; originally published in 1975). It was also concerned with the prevention of sexual problems and the strengthening of marriages. The second way that Masters and Johnson wanted to tackle sexual inadequacy was through sex therapy. They intended right from the start of their research to use their data on human sexual functioning as a foundation on which to develop (like medicine) rational and effective treatment interventions for people with sexual dysfunctions (Masters and Johnson 1970, 1; Masters et al 1985, 21).

These interventions — educational and therapeutic — would also have a commercial side to them, and this fact did not escape Masters and Johnson's attention. While they operated primarily in terms of a professed concern for the well-being of the sexually inadequate, rather than self-interest, they were nevertheless aware of the potential size of the markets for sexual information and therapy. They noted Golden's observation, for example, that selling sexual information was very profitable and that the demand for basic sexual information was part of the appeal of pornography (Masters and Johnson 1966, v).

Masters and Johnson were later able to cash-in on their authority, expertise and research. They partly funded their work over a long period from the sale of books, information and advice. Three years after the closure of their institute in 1994, Johnson also 'invested her name and expertise' in a commercial mail-order business called the Virginia Johnson Masters Learning Center (Levins 1997, F1). The centre aimed for an economic return from the sale of printed material and audio cassettes to those experiencing dissatisfaction, dysfunction and disorder. Johnson was reported as saying drily 'I did non-profit long enough' (Levins 1997, F1).

Masters and Johnson (1970, 369) would have also anticipated a fairly large market for sex therapy services given that they believed half the marriages in the United States were sexually dysfunctional or would be so in the near future. Presumably, they understood what market size would mean for those able to establish themselves as the foremost authorities on sex and innovators of a radically new approach to sex therapy.

The third reason for the Sex Research Project was that Masters hoped his dispassionate scientific work would help to free the study of sex from the fear, ignorance, prejudice and political pressure which had stifled previous sex research. He believed that these constraints were primarily responsible for the dearth of reliable scientific information on human sexual response. Reducing these constraints was an important priority not only to further his own work but to make sex research a less hazardous and more productive venture for his contemporaries and successors. Masters and Johnson (1966, vii) later portrayed their work as a 'faltering step... toward an open-door policy' on sex research, and they thanked Alfred Kinsey for having opened the door for them.

FUNDING AND LOCATION OF THE RESEARCH

In 1954, Masters was funded for the first two years of his research by Washington University. After the funding ceased, Masters supported his project with small grants from individuals and a larger grant of $14,000 from a St. Louis businessman. In 1958, the National Institute of Health, a part of the United States Public Health Service, provided Masters and Johnson with a grant of $25,000 a year for four years (Belliveau and Richter 1971, 20). Since then, Masters and Johnson have been funded from Masters' gynaecological practice, book sales, workshop and clinic fees, local companies, small philanthropic organisations, individual donations and the Playboy Foundation (Brecher and Brecher 1967, 43; Belliveau and Richter 1971, 21; Irvine 1990a, 80). Mackinnon (1987, 143, 261) points out that Playboy alone had given Masters and Johnson over $300,000 by November 1979.

The project was based at the medical school until 1964 when Masters set up his own Reproductive Biology Research Foundation in a building near the university (Brecher and Brecher 1967, 43). The foundation moved again to new premises in the late 1970s. At this time it had twenty-five members of staff and a long waiting list of patients (Heidenry 1997, 277). The name of the foundation was changed to the Masters and Johnson Institute in 1979. This was to celebrate the twenty-fifth anniversary of their research. 'The original name, chosen to sound nonthreatening, had proven too clumsy and difficult to remember' (Irvine 1990a, 80), and the new name was intended to boost their efforts at fund raising (Heidenry 1997, 289). By the end of 1994, however, the Institute had closed. The main reasons for the closure were a 'chronic lack of funding', dwindling numbers of patients, Masters' deteriorating health (from over-work and Parkinson's disease), and the inability of Masters and Johnson to agree on the future direction of the Institute and the appointment of a successor. Johnson, who is now retired, retained most of the archives of the Institute after its closure. She is reported to be working on a 'tell-all' memoir of her experiences (Heidenry 1997, 394, 396). Masters died from Parkinson's disease on 16 February, 2001. He was 85 (Dead or Alive? 2001).

MAIN RESEARCH QUESTIONS AND THE
INFLUENCE OF SCIENTIFIC MEDICINE

Masters set out to answer two main questions in his laboratory research on human sexual response: 'What happens to the human male and female as they respond to effective sexual stimulation? Why do men and women behave as they do when responding to effective sexual stimulation?' (Masters and Johnson 1966, 10).

In his attempt to answer these questions, Masters was strongly influenced by the practice of scientific medicine. In Western industrialised societies, the medical profession has historically been the most successful group in determining which conditions represent health or illness (even if they have not always been unchallenged). Medicine's authority over these areas rests, in part, on claims that medical knowledge is based on scientific research, particularly in disciplines like microbiology, chemistry and physics (Jefferys 1988, 225). The association of medicine with the natural sciences has promoted the belief that medical knowledge is scientific, objective and value free (Roach Anleu 1991, 10). A key aim of medical science is to provide data on normal anatomy and physiology so that deviations from the norm can be identified and appropriately treated.

Medicine provided the model Masters would follow in terms of his aim of establishing on a scientific basis the normal physiology of human sexual functioning. This norm would be crucial in paving the way for and legitimising the later development of his and Johnson's sex therapy program. Deviations from normal sexual functioning would constitute the sexual dysfunctions which sex therapists could identify, investigate and treat in order to secure a return to normal sexual functioning. Scientific legitimacy was also important for two other reasons. Firstly, it helped sexologists like Masters and Johnson to challenge the knowledge claims of psychoanalysts who were their main competitors for the sex therapy market. Secondly, the mantle of science helped to make sex research more publicly respectable and viable (by modelling it on scientific medicine) in a climate of spirited opposition from individuals and groups with strong moral and religious views on its appropriateness (Masters and Johnson 1970; Masters et al 1985, 21; Bejin 1986a).

INITIAL RESEARCH WITH PROSTITUTES

To carry out his research, Masters needed research participants. He initially decided to study female and male prostitutes because he thought that non-prostitute volunteers would be too difficult to obtain for his research. He was also attracted to research with prostitutes because they were available for money, because they would be knowledgeable and cooperative subjects, and because he thought he might discover things from them which were not in the scientific literature. Washington University's Chancellor, Ethan She-pley, gave Masters permission to study prostitutes provided he worked with a review board including the St. Louis police commissioner, the publisher of the *St. Louis Globe-Democrat,* and the head of the St. Louis Roman Catholic Archdiocese (Heidenry 1997, 25; Kolodny 2001, 274).

The police commissioner put Masters in touch with some prostitutes, and arranged for him to watch them with their clients from small voy-eurs' booths in a succession of brothels. Masters conducted his research with prostitutes for eighteen months in brothels in Canada, Mexico, the Midwest and the West Coast. He studied a wide range of sexual experi-ence, including all the variations of sexual intercourse, fetishes, oral sex and anal sex. He interviewed female prostitutes after their sexual activity and examined their swollen genitals. He also enquired about their sexual techniques, and a range of sexual phenomena including vaginal orgasm, orgasm without genital stimulation and multiple orgasm (Heidenry 1997, 25). In the first twenty months of his research, Masters interviewed a total of 118 female and 27 male prostitutes about their occupations, sociosexual and medical histories (Masters and Johnson 1966, 10).

After Masters had learned everything he could from his research in the brothels, he prepared for the laboratory stage of his research. He quietly opened a clinic with an office and laboratories on the upper floor of a maternity hospital linked to Washington University (Heidenry 1997, 25–6). He then selected eight female prostitutes and three male prostitutes for laboratory study. The study of their anatomies and physiological responses provided a trial run and necessary refinements for the later research proj-ect. The prostitutes also provided Masters with invaluable advice about sexual techniques. They described different ways of increasing or moderat-ing sexual arousal and demonstrated enormous variations in their methods of stimulation. Many of these techniques were later found to have direct application in sex therapy and were incorporated into clinical research (Masters and Johnson 1966, 10; Belliveau and Richter 1971, 25).

Irvine (1990a, 82) has emphasised that the prostitutes who collabo-rated in this early research can be regarded as 'sexologists in their own right.' They knew more about sexual functioning and sexual technique than Masters and his colleagues. 'Without their collaboration, it is doubt-ful that Masters and Johnson's research would have achieved the degree of sophistication it did, at least within such a short time frame' (Irvine 1990a, 82).

Ultimately, however, Masters did not use the physiological research data provided by these participants. He thought that long term study of this group would be difficult because many were transient residents of the local area. In addition, he reported that many of the prostitutes had vary-ing degrees of pelvic pathology, including chronic congestion of the pelvic region. Masters believed that this was caused by frequent sexual arousal without orgasm. He thought the pelvic pathology would prevent him from establishing a baseline of normal anatomic data in his research (Masters and Johnson 1966, 11; Belliveau and Richter 1971, 25).

Masters' decision to exclude the prostitutes on this latter ground is questionable. Firstly, although his complaint seems to be directed more at the female rather than the male prostitutes, it is not clear why healthy male (or female) prostitutes should also be excluded on this ground. Secondly, he apparently assumed, in any case, that the female prostitutes were unlike the 'average woman' who 'does not frequently experience sexual arousal without having orgasm' (O'Connell Davidson and Layder 1994, 152). Yet Kinsey et al's (1953) research casts some doubt on this. Published just one year before Masters' research began, Kinsey et al (1953, 375) found that between 36 and 44% of women in their sample experienced orgasm in only some of their marital coitus.

> About one-third of those females had responded only a small part of the time, another third had responded more or less half of the time, and the other third had responded a major portion of the time, even though it was not a hundred per cent of the time. (Kinsey et al 1953, 375)

The final service that the prostitutes provided to Masters was their advice that non-prostitute volunteers might not be too difficult to obtain, and that he should hire a female research assistant to help him work with female research volunteers (Brecher 1970, 296; Belliveau and Richter 1971, 25).

HIRING OF VIRGINIA JOHNSON AND SELECTION OF NEW RESEARCH PARTICIPANTS

In order to attract non-prostitute volunteers, Masters publicised his need for research participants throughout Washington University (Brecher 1970, 296). It was during the phase of recruiting volunteers in 1957 that Virginia Johnson (1925-) came to work with Masters. He wanted an intelligent assistant, aged in her 'late twenties or early thirties', who was 'married and divorced' with at least one child, and who could 'work well with people'. Masters thought it most important that she 'knew where babies came from' and did not have a 'professional virgin psyche' (Belliveau and Richter 1971, 15; 'Playboy Interview: Masters and Johnson' 1976, 133; Irvine 1990a, 79).

Johnson was a twice divorced mother of two who was looking for work when she registered for a job with Washington University's placement bureau. She had no degree but had worked as a secretary, and was pursuing a singing career on an amateur basis (Heidenry 1997, 27). She was looking for a job that would earn her enough money to live on 'without boring her to death' and became involved with Masters' project 'by total coincidence' (Murray 1976, 200). She said, 'I'd never in a million years have chosen this particular work' (Murray 1976, 200). Masters interviewed her in December 1956 and she started the following January. He 'was astute enough to realize her personable manner ideally complemented his own stern, circumspect bearing' (Heidenry 1997, 27). Johnson promised herself that she would quit her position after ten years and resume her singing career (Heidenry 1997, 27). In fact, she ended up working with Masters for thirty-five years until 1992. They also married in 1971 (Masters' second marriage) and remained married until an amicable divorce in 1993 ('Sex researchers Masters, Johnson granted divorce' 1993; Nemy 1994; Heidenry 1997, 168).

Masters did not recruit Johnson as his academic equal. He had specified that applicants for the position as his assistant should not have a post-graduate degree. He apparently feared that his assistant's involvement in sex research might lead to the loss of her degree and damage to her professional career. He may also not have wanted an assistant with graduate school theories which would interfere with his own (Heidenry 1997, 26–7). Thus, while Johnson later called herself a psychologist, she did not have a degree, and her highest educational qualification was a high school diploma (Szasz 1981, 28). It seems that Masters primarily chose Johnson for her ability to work long hours with him (hence she could not be married), her ability to relate to people, especially female research participants, and her ability to 'get the best out of them' (Belliveau and Richter 1971, 15; Murray 1976, 199; Irvine 1990a, 80). Masters did ensure though that Johnson got equal credit for their work both professionally and publicly (Nemy 1994).

People who volunteered for Masters and Johnson's research had to undergo a screening interview and physical examination before they could be accepted. The interview was to ascertain the willingness of volunteers to participate in the research, their capacity for sexual response, and their ability to articulate in fine detail the nature of their sexual responses. The physical examination was to establish that the reproductive systems of volunteers were anatomically 'normal.' While people with 'normally' occurring variations in reproductive anatomy were included in the research, people with grossly abnormal reproductive systems were excluded. Masters and Johnson (1966, 12) did not define what they meant by 'grossly abnormal reproductive viscera.' Volunteers also had to have a 'positive history of masturbatory and coital orgasmic experience' before they could be accepted (Masters and Johnson 1966, 311). Masters stated that 'If you are going to find out what happens, obviously, you must work with those to whom it happens' ('Playboy Interview: Masters and Johnson' 1976, 129). If participants could not reach orgasm during coitus and masturbation while being observed in the laboratory, they were excluded from the research (Brecher 1970, 298). This apparently did not include individuals who experienced intermittent performance failures (Masters and Johnson 1966, 312–15). In addition, Masters and Johnson (1966, 12) excluded any volunteers with 'sociosexual aberrancy.' They did not define the meaning of this term either.

Masters and Johnson (1966, 13) finally chose 694 research participants from a population of 1273 people who had been interviewed. The 694 people comprised 276 married couples and 142 unmarried individuals (although 98 individuals from this latter group had previously been married) (Masters and Johnson 1966, 15). In all, a total of 382 women participated in the research with ages ranging from 18–78 years but with most participants (84%) between the ages of 18 and 40 years. The female sample included seven women who participated in studies of the artificial vagina's sexual response, and six women who acted as research participants in a study of sexual response during pregnancy. A total of 312 men participated in the research, their ages ranging from 21–89 years but with most participants (74%) between the ages of 21 and 40 years. The male sample included both men who were uncircumcised (35 individuals) and men who were circumcised (the remainder) (Masters and Johnson 1966, 12–18).

Masters and Johnson's (1966, 8) sample was not representative of U.S. society. The size of the sample was statistically inadequate mainly due to insufficient research funding (Masters and Johnson 1966, 19). The sample was also a selective one in many ways. Most of the research participants came from the surrounding academic community. They were predominantly white, heterosexual, of average or above average 'intelligence,' highly educated, of high socioeconomic status and between the ages of 18 and 40 (Masters and Johnson 1966).

There are a number of reasons why Masters and Johnson (1966, 12) selected this sample and deliberately weighted it toward people of higher than average 'intelligence' and socioeconomic status. Firstly, the volunteers were regarded as more 'respectable' people than the prostitutes who had participated in Masters' early research. These 'respectable' volunteers would not attract the same level of censure or opprobrium to the research project as the prostitutes. Brecher (1970, 295) points out, for example, that when Masters' research first became publicly known, his 'use of prostitutes became the subject of snide remarks and leers.' Some critics insisted that the research with prostitutes was worthless and that Masters had demeaned himself by contact with them. Secondly, the 'respectable' volunteers were readily available for Masters and Johnson's research. They came primarily from the surrounding academic community, they had free time to participate in the research, and they could participate over a sustained period if necessary (Robinson 1976, 134). Finally, the selection bias toward higher 'intelligence' and socioeconomic status served to make the research population socially similar to the researchers. This meant that the volunteers would be more likely to appreciate the significance of the research, that they would be easier to work with, and that it would be easier to elicit information from them (Irvine 1990a, 83). For example,

Masters and Johnson (1966, 12) had stressed in the initial intake interviews that research participants had to be able to describe in fine detail the nature of their sexual responses.

The lack of a representative sample, however, meant that Masters and Johnson were unable to answer one of their two original research questions.

> The question of why men and women respond as they do to effective sexual stimulation is not answered in this text. Neither the laboratory-study subject nor the clinical research populations are sufficiently representative of the general population to allow definitive conclusions to be supported from behavioral material drawn from these groups and reported in the text. (Masters and Johnson 1966, 8)

Masters and Johnson assumed, however, that their non-representative sample would not affect their ability to answer their first research question concerning what happens to men and women as they respond to sexual stimulation. They defended their narrow sample by emphasising that their research concerned physiology and not psychology ('Playboy Interview: Masters and Johnson' 1976, 140). Their defence relied on essentialist assumptions about the 'primacy and universality of the human body' and a lack of regard for possible mediating effects of social backgrounds and characteristics (Irvine 1990a, 84). Brecher and Brecher (1967, 60) epitomised this defence of Masters and Johnson with their statement that 'The higher-average educational level of the women volunteers is hardly likely to affect the acidity of their vaginal fluids.'

Masters and Johnson (1966), however, did not test the validity of this assumption, and as mentioned in chapter 3, there is research which demonstrates that the social can affect the biological. It could even be argued that Masters and Johnson were partially aware of this even though they did not fully explore its implications for their own research. For example, they excluded prostitutes from their research partly because many of them had chronic pelvic congestion which might have affected their sexual response. Yet the very reason for this pelvic congestion had to do with the social context of the prostitutes' work in which they experienced frequent sexual arousal without orgasm. It is also interesting to note that Masters and Johnson later abandoned their essentialist defence when they replicated their research with a homosexual population in order to discover whether homosexuals and heterosexuals have different physiological responses to sexual stimulation (Irvine 1990a, 84). Perhaps, not surprisingly, Masters and Johnson's (1979, 226) conclusion, published in their book *Homosexuality in Perspective,* was that 'no real difference exists between homosexual men and women and heterosexual men and women in their physiologic capacity to respond to similar sexual stimuli'.

ORIENTATION TO THE LABORATORY

Once the volunteers were selected they entered an orientation program. They were taken to a moderate-sized laboratory room with light green walls and no windows. The back of the room had a small one-way mirror which enabled staff to carry out observations from an adjacent room. However, this was rarely used by Masters and Johnson. They showed the research participants where the mirror was and how it could be blocked if people wanted privacy. The researchers preferred to build up trust with the participants, and to help them become accustomed gradually to the researchers' presence during sexual activity. Inside the laboratory itself was a bed, floodlights, colour movie cameras, a transparent plastic phallus with a light source and camera inside, and various scientific instruments which allowed Masters and Johnson to record subjects' heart rates, blood pressure, respiratory rates, brain-wave patterns and other bodily activity during sexual arousal. The temperature, humidity and lighting in the room were all controllable (Belliveau and Richter 1971, 27; Heidenry 1997, 26–9).

After being introduced to the laboratory and its equipment, research participants were allowed time to adjust to their surroundings. Sexual activity was encouraged, at first in private, and later with the researchers present until the volunteers felt comfortable with the environment, and confident that they could sexually perform. The laboratory research began once the volunteers were regarded as properly acclimatised (Masters and Johnson 1966, 22–3). 'Couples were ... told ahead of time that they would be observed during sexual activity not only by therapists but possibly by assistants, artists and cameramen' (Belliveau and Richter 1971, 27).

Volunteers were also paid a small but unspecified amount of money for their participation (Belliveau and Richter 1971, 26; 'Playboy Interview: Masters and Johnson' 1976, 141). The payments were similar to customary payments made for other types of laboratory research, and were intended to offset costs of participation, such as cab fares and baby-sitters. They also provided some monetary incentive for couples needing extra money, and were an inducement to volunteers to keep their appointments punctually (Brecher and Brecher 1968, 68–9).

NATURE AND DURATION OF THE SEX RESEARCH

Masters and Johnson sought to protect the volunteers' privacy by working odd hours, and by having staff patrol the hallway to ensure that volunteers were not seen entering or exiting the laboratory (Heidenry 1997, 26, 28). Masters and Johnson (1966, 21, 54, 67) reported that during the course of the laboratory studies, research participants engaged in a variety of sexual activities including manual masturbation; masturbation with a mechanical vibrator; coitus with the female partner on her back, in a knee-chest position or with the man on his back; vaginal intercourse with a plastic phallus controlled by the woman while on her back or in a knee-chest position; and sexual stimulation of the woman's breasts alone without additional genital stimulation. The researchers apparently also collected data on other types of sexual acts, including variations of heterosexual and homosexual intercourse, but this was withheld from publication to increase the acceptability of their work (Masters and Johnson 1966, 22; Heidenry 1997, 36). During these sexual activities, there were usually at least two observers in the room, in addition to one or two physiologists, who would occasionally be present to monitor the recording equipment or operate the cameras (Heidenry 1997, 30). 'Many experiments were filmed' (Belliveau and Richter 1971, 27). However, the camera never filmed people's faces or entire bodies. It focused only on one part of the body at a time in order to record specific physiological changes there, such as changes to skin colour or vaginal lubrication ('Playboy Interview: Masters and Johnson' 1976, 137).

Masters and Johnson themselves comprised the basic research team but they always made sure both sexes were represented in the laboratory. This was to ensure the comfort and security of the volunteers and to help them adjust to their environment. The researchers structured the laboratory sessions so that their own presence was as unobtrusive as possible. They tried to behave in a calm, and matter-of-fact way and set out to make the research seem like a routine hour in the laboratory rather than a sexual spectacle in front of an audience (Brecher and Brecher 1968, 64–5). Technicians and volunteers also distinguished between 'work time' and 'non-work time' in the laboratory so that when sessions were over people would cover up or turn away in order to preserve some privacy ('Playboy Interview: Masters and Johnson': 1976, 143).

Masters and Johnson were almost completely consumed by their work. They worked gruelling seven-day weeks, and from July 1, 1954, Masters did not take a day off for seventeen years, even working through Christmas and New Year holidays (Nemy 1994; Heidenry 1997, 28). Over an eleven year period from 1954 they observed, measured and recorded the physical details of human sexual response under scientific laboratory conditions. In their work, they give a strong impression of being empiricists, busily gathering the 'facts' about human sexual physiology in an atheoretical way (Bancroft 1989, 462). By 1965, they estimated that their volunteers had collectively experienced at least 10,000 orgasms (Masters and Johnson 1966, 15). Their research led to the publication of various scholarly articles (see, for example, Masters and Johnson 1963; 1965a; 1965b; 1965c) and their famous book *Human Sexual Response* in 1966. After completing their physiology research in 1970, their laboratory was dismantled (Irvine 1990a, 81).

THE HUMAN SEXUAL RESPONSE CYCLE

Masters and Johnson's (1966) major research finding was that the sexual responses of males and females are so similar that they can be understood as occurring within a single human sexual response cycle. This cycle has four stages: excitement, plateau, orgasm and resolution.

1. Excitement

The excitement stage is a person's first reaction to sexual stimulation. Excitement can occur as the result of physical and/or psychological stimulation (Masters and Johnson 1966, 5–6). In females, the first sign of sexual excitement is vaginal lubrication which starts to appear within ten to thirty seconds after sexual stimulation begins (Masters and Johnson 1966, 69). As excitement continues, myotonia (neuromuscular tension) causes the inner two-thirds of the normally touching vaginal walls to become wider and longer, and the cervix and uterus are pulled upward (Masters and Johnson 1966, 71, 82, 112). The labia majora flatten and separate, and the labia minora increase in diameter (Masters and Johnson 1966, 38–41). The clitoris increases in size and is brought into closer contact with the clitoral foreskin (Masters and Johnson 1966, 48–9). Nipple erection typically occurs, the veins in the breasts may become more noticeable and the breasts may slightly increase in size (Masters and Johnson 1966, 28–9).

In males, the first and most obvious sign of sexual arousal is erection of the penis. This can occur within seconds of sexual stimulation. As a result of vasocongestion (the swelling of blood vessels), the penis increases in size and hardness and becomes erect. As excitation continues, the scrotal skin tenses and thickens and the testes are partially elevated toward the body (Masters and Johnson 1966, 182, 204–6).

2. Plateau

In the plateau stage, sexual arousal is basically intensified beyond excitement levels to a point where it could lead to orgasm if stimulation continued. In females, vasocongestion causes tissues in the outer third of the vagina to swell in a process called the 'orgasmic platform.' This swelling narrows the size of the vaginal opening by more than 30% (Masters and Johnson 1966, 76). The inner two-thirds of the vagina increases slightly in width and depth and the uterus reaches a position of full elevation. The production of vaginal lubrication slows down (Masters and Johnson 1966, 76–7, 112). The labia minora increase by two or three times in diameter and protrude through and separate the labia majora. This makes the vaginal opening more accessible (Masters and Johnson 1966, 40–1). Once this has occurred, the minor labia dramatically change colour. In women who have never been pregnant, the colour of the labia minora varies from pink to bright red, while in women who have been pregnant, the colour ranges from 'bright red to a deep wine color' (Masters and Johnson 1966, 41). No women were seen achieving orgasm without first exhibiting these minor-labial colour changes (Masters and Johnson 1966, 42). If effective sexual stimulation continues once this colour change has occurred then orgasm will inevitably follow (Masters and Johnson 1966, 41).

The clitoris pulls back from its 'normal pudendal-overhang' position and retracts against the pubic bone. Any part of the clitoral glans which normally extends beyond the clitoral hood in a sexually unaroused condition is hidden under the protective foreskin. As the clitoris retracts, the length of the clitoral shaft is reduced by at least 50% (Masters and Johnson 1966, 51).

The areola of the female breast continues to swell so that the earlier nipple erection is less pronounced and the breasts of women who have not suckled children may increase in size by 20 to 25%. For women who have suckled children, there are not the same marked increases in breast size (Masters and Johnson 1966, 29). Late in the excitement stage or early in the plateau stage a reddish measles-like rash or 'sex-flush' appears in about 75% of women. It usually begins under the breast bone and extends rapidly to the breasts and chest. It may also develop in other parts of the body including the face, shoulders, back, thighs and buttocks (Masters and Johnson 1966, 31–2). Heart rate, blood pressure and myotonia also increase during the plateau stage and breathing becomes faster (Masters and Johnson 1966, 32–6).

In males, the coronal ridge of the glans penis increases slightly in diameter and the colour of the glans may deepen to a reddish-purple colour as a result of vasocongestion (Masters and Johnson 1966, 183–4). The testes continue to elevate until they rest against the perineum. If effective sexual stimulation continues then orgasm will be sure to follow. If the testes do not elevate, at least partially, then males will not fully achieve ejaculation (Masters and Johnson 1966, 207–8). Vasocongestion also causes the testes to increase in size by between 50 to 100% when compared to their unstimulated state (Masters and Johnson 1966, 208). Frequently two or three drops of clear pre-ejaculatory fluid emerge from the tip of the penis. The fluid is believed to come from Cowper's glands and sometimes carries live sperm (Masters and Johnson 1966, 210–11). About one-quarter of men develop a sex flush similar to that described for women (Masters and Johnson 1966, 172–3). Heart rate, blood pressure and myotonia also increases during the plateau stage and breathing becomes faster (Masters and Johnson 1966, 173–6).

3. Orgasm

If effective sexual stimulation continues through the plateau stage then orgasm will occur. During orgasm there is a massive release of the muscle tension which has built up during the excitement and plateau stages. This is accompanied by intensely pleasurable sensations. Orgasm is the shortest stage of the sexual response cycle and lasts for just a few seconds (Masters and Johnson 1966, 6; Masters et al 1985, 86).

In females, orgasm is characterised by a series of involuntary muscle contractions which occur simultaneously in the outer third of the vagina, the uterus and the anal sphincter. The contractions occur at 0.8 second intervals and the number may vary from a minimum of three to five to a maximum of ten to fifteen depending on the intensity of the orgasmic experience. The contractions diminish in intensity and duration as the orgasm continues and the interval between contractions also becomes less regular (Masters and Johnson 1966, 34, 77–8, 116).

In males, unlike females, the physiological expression of orgasm occurs in two main stages. In the first stage of male orgasm, semen is expelled via a series of involuntary contractions from the vas deferens, prostate and seminal vesicles into the bulb at the base of the urethra. In the second stage of orgasm, the contractions of the prostate, urethra and penis propel the seminal fluid through the urethra and out of the urethral meatus at the tip of the penis. During ejaculation the sphincter of the urinary bladder is closed so that seminal fluid cannot enter the bladder nor urine escape and mix with the semen. The rhythmic contractions which occur during male orgasm also include the anus and, as in women, occur at 0.8 second intervals. After the first three or four contractions, the interval between contractions increases and their intensity weakens (Masters and Johnson 1966, 173–4, 212–13; Masters et al 1985, 90).

4. Resolution

After individuals have experienced orgasm, they enter the resolution stage. In this stage there is essentially a reversal of the physiological changes which characterised the excitement and plateau stages as the body returns to a sexually unstimulated state. Vasocongestion dissipates as blood is released from congested blood vessels and neuromuscular tension subsides. The time taken to reach complete resolution is about the same as the time spent in the excitement and plateau stages. If sexual excitement has been intense and prolonged, however, and if orgasm has not occurred, then it may take much longer to achieve full resolution (Masters and Johnson 1966, 6–7, 283–5, 300).

In females, swelling in the outer third of the vagina decreases, the uterus descends to its normal resting place, the vivid colour of the labia minora disappears, the vagina begins to contract in both length and width, the clitoris loses its tumescence and returns to its normal 'pudendal overhang position', breast size is reduced, the areolae and nipples lose their swelling and the sex flush disappears (Masters and Johnson 1966, 30–1, 42, 52–3, 78–80).

In males, resolution is characterised by a two stage detumescence of the erect penis. Firstly, orgasmic contractions cause a rapid pumping of blood from the penis so that its size is reduced to about 50% larger than its unstimulated condition. Secondly, there is a more gradual process of blood flow from the penis until it returns to its unstimulated size and shape. The testes decrease in size, move away from the body and descend into the scrotum. The tenseness and congestion of the scrotum dissipates and the characteristic folding of its skin returns (Masters and Johnson 1966, 185–7, 205–6, 209; Masters et al 1985, 93).

According to Masters and Johnson (1966, 6–7), there is one major difference between females and males in the resolution stage. Females have the ability while experiencing resolution to return to the orgasmic stage if effective sexual stimulation recommences. This capacity is particularly evident if stimulation recommences while females are still in the plateau stage of sexual tension. This means that females have the physiological potential to experience multiple orgasms: a series of separate and complete orgasms within a short time of each other without falling below the plateau stage of sexual arousal (Masters et al 1985, 92).

Males, on the other hand, enter a unique refractory period during resolution which females do not. This period begins immediately after ejaculation and lasts until male sexual tensions are reduced to low levels of excitement stage response (Masters and Johnson 1966, 283). This period is variable and may last anywhere from a couple of minutes to many hours. The refractory period can vary between males and even for the same male in different sexual situations. During the refractory period further sexual stimulation to orgasm is physiologically impossible. Effective restimulation can only begin once the refractory period is over. This means that males are not physiologically capable of experiencing multiple orgasms if this term is defined in the same way as for females (Masters and Johnson 1966, 6–7, 283–4; Masters et al 1985, 92).

PUBLICATION AND RECEPTION OF *HUMAN SEXUAL RESPONSE*

Masters and Johnson initially kept their research as secret as possible by gaining press cooperation not to publicise information about their project. Masters also ensured secrecy by personally selecting the board members of the Reproductive Biology Research Foundation. These members included Washington University's Chancellor, the police commissioner and the local newspaper publisher. Masters and Johnson believed that premature publicity could seriously threaten the viability of their project. This strategy worked for about ten years. However, in 1964, the psychoanalyst Leslie Farber published a stinging attack on their work after reading an early article they had published in a medical journal. His attack focused widespread public attention on their work and Masters and Johnson felt under pressure to publish their research in order to provide an accurate account to the public (Farber 1968; 'Playboy Interview: Masters and Johnson' 1976, 135; Irvine 1990a, 81).

This account took the form of a book called *Human Sexual Response*. It has been described as one of 'the worst written books in the English language' (Robinson 1976, 123) and as 'an almost impenetrable thicket of Latinate medicalese' ('Playboy Interview: Masters and Johnson' 1976, 129). Masters and Johnson's writing style, though, was no accident. It was designed to minimise the possibility of negative public reaction. According to Masters:

> Every effort was made to make this book as pedantic and obtuse as possible and, may I say in all modesty, I think we succeeded admirably. Although we were specifically writing a textbook for the biological and behavioral professions, we were all aware that the text would be dissected paragraph by paragraph by others, and that if one line, or even a suggestion of 'pornography' could be established in any context, we would have had to face a holocaust. (Irvine 1990a, 81)

Human Sexual Response was published in April 1966 by the medical division of the staid publishing house Little, Brown and Company. They issued the book in 'a plain brown wrapper' and did not spend any money on trade advertising. The initial print run of 15,000 copies was sold out even before the official publishing date ('Playboy Interview: Masters and Johnson' 1976, 129). Even though *Human Sexual Response* was a medical book it quickly reached 'number two position on the *New York Times* non-fiction bestseller list' (Belliveau and Richter 1971, 59) and remained on the *Publishers' Weekly's* best-seller list for six months. By 1968, it had sold over 300,000 copies at ten dollars per copy and continued to sell 2,000 to 3,000 copies a month. It was also translated into nine foreign languages. By comparison, the average medical text at that time sold only 10,000 copies in total ('Playboy Interview: Masters and Johnson' 1976, 129). Another 500,000 paperback copies of Ruth and Edward Brecher's account of *Human Sexual Response* were sold by 1969, and their book, too, was translated into nine different languages (Brecher 1970, 280).

With the publication of *Human Sexual Response,* Masters and Johnson became world famous virtually overnight. On the day of publication, newspapers in many countries reported on their research and frequently provided follow-up stories (Brecher 1970, 280). Magazines such as *Time* and *Newsweek* featured their research and tens of millions of readers learned about their work from this type of exposure (Irvine 1990a, 68). 'Not since the Kinsey reports had sex research made such a stir in the world' (Brecher 1970, 280).

The reaction to *Human Sexual Response* was generally favourable. Masters said that of 'approximately 700 reviews in both the medical and the lay press' only about 10% were critical in the sense that reviewers thought 'the work should not have been done' ('Playboy Interview: Masters and Johnson' 1976, 135). The actual findings themselves attracted relatively little criticism. Belliveau and Richter (1971, 64), for example, stated that since *Human Sexual Response* was published 'there has been no serious scientific challenge to it. The findings...have become widely accepted.' *MD* magazine, in one of its editorials, wrote that the:

> best measure of the study's professional acceptance...is that 25 medical schools have instituted courses in the physiology of human sexual response, and 14 more are beginning in the coming semester. The text in use is their book; there is no other. ('Playboy Interview: Masters and Johnson' 1976, 131)

Masters later added that there were hardly any medical courses on human sexual response prior to 1964 but that since then 'somewhere between 40 and 50 medical schools — out of a possible 92 — have begun teaching courses in sexual response. This represents a real revolution in medical education' ('Playboy Interview: Masters and Johnson' 1976, 162).

Another significant indicator of *Human Sexual Response*'s professional acceptance is that the centrepiece of that work — the human sexual response cycle — was incorporated (in an amended form) into the American Psychiatric Association's *Diagnostic and Statistical Manual of Mental Disorders (DSM-III* 1980). This cycle is used as the norm of sexual functioning from which sexual dysfunctions are distinguished. The *DSM-III* (1980) contains a sexual response cycle with four stages: appetitive, excitement, orgasm and resolution. The appetitive stage was added to Masters and Johnson's model when the sex therapist Helen Kaplan (1979, xviii) argued that sexual desire should be included for 'conceptual completeness and clinical effectiveness.' The *DSM-III* (1980) also modified the original Masters and Johnson model by collapsing the excitement and plateau stages into a single excitement stage. Masters and Johnson's research, however, remained the major underpinning of the model and they 'are cited in the DSM footnotes as the primary source' (Tiefer 1991a, 12). The same model was retained in the *DSM-III-R* (1987), the *DSM-IV* (1994), and the *DSM-IV-TR* (2000). In the latter two editions, however, the 'Appetitive' phase of the sexual response cycle was renamed the 'Desire' phase (American Psychiatric Association 1994; 2000).

Even twenty-one years after *Human Sexual Response* was published, Stephen Goettsch (1987) could find little, if any, criticism of Masters and Johnson's (1966) research findings when he reviewed eight contemporary textbooks on human sexuality. He wrote, for example, that 'Every text presents Masters and Johnson's (1966) sexual response cycle, frequently without criticism or contradictory research' (Goettsch 1987, 327). The uncritical acceptance of Masters and Johnson's model of the sexual response cycle was still evident more than thirty years after *Human Sexual Response* was published (Tiefer 1996, 259; Goren 2003, 494).

Masters and Johnson's (1966) work also proved to be popular with many feminists. Its publication coincided with the second wave of feminism (Tiefer 1991a, 6), and it was seen as not only challenging the sexual myths of the past but providing a 'positive assertion of female sexuality in contemporary western (sic) thought' (Segal 1983, 33). One of the major findings of *Human Sexual Response* challenged the Freudian view that clitoral and vaginal orgasms were distinct anatomical entities and that clitoral orgasms were 'immature' in comparison with their vaginal counterparts. Masters and Johnson (1966, 66) found that there was no essential physiological difference between a clitoral and vaginal orgasm. They wrote that the physiological responses of the internal organs of the female pelvis to effective sexual stimulation are the same irrespective of whether a woman receives stimulation via her mons, clitoris, vagina or other erogenous parts of her body. 'This finding proved tremendously liberating for scores of women who felt inadequate, incomplete, or immature if they had been unable to experience the so-called vaginal orgasm during intercourse' (Leiblum and Pervin 1980, 13). Some feminists went even further and argued that if the notion of a distinct vaginal orgasm was a myth then in anatomical terms men's penises could be regarded as irrelevant for female sexual pleasure. Anne Koedt (1973, 205–6), for example, thought that women could just as easily find sexual pleasure with other women, as with men, and that men would fear becoming 'sexually expendable.'

Feminists also tended to see Masters and Johnson's (1966) research as liberating to women by challenging the view that women were asexual or had a weaker and inferior sexual 'nature' than men. Masters and Johnson's research emphasised that women actually have a greater physiological capacity for sex than men, and are capable of multiple orgasms while men are limited by the onset of a refractory period. Feminists, such as Mary Jane Sherfey (1972, 112), seized on this finding to argue that 'To all intents and purposes, *the human female is sexually insatiable*' (emphasis in original). Tiefer (1991a, 7) concluded that 'These "scientific facts" affirmed women's political claims for sexual pleasure and entitlement and thus feminists saw sexologists as allies in their struggle against ignorance and sexism.'

When Masters and Johnson's (1966) research was criticised, the criticism focused much more on their research methods than their actual findings (Gagnon 1975, 137). Dr. Leslie Farber, who launched the initial attack on Masters and Johnson, set the trend for many of the subsequent criticisms. He accused Masters and Johnson of mechanising and dehumanising sex, of selecting atypical research subjects and of neglecting the psychological dimension of sex (Brecher and Brecher 1968, 323). To talk about sex with people outside clinical settings, as Kinsey had done, 'was one thing but the observation of sexual behavior and its measurement through dials and indicators seemed a final sacrilege' (Gagnon 1975, 137). Critics wondered 'what kind of mind could have devised such an experiment, or, worse, what kind of person could be so depraved as to volunteer for it' (Ehrenreich, Hess and Jacobs 1987, 66). Critics tended to see the research as pornographic and as representing the final disenchantment of the sexual. The psychoanalyst Natalie Shainess, for example, believed that Masters and Johnson had discharged 'a pipeline of pornographic sewage...into the vital heart of our life,' 'thingified sex,' 'trivialized it...[and] trampled on the ultimate mystery of life' (Ehrenreich et al 1987, 66).

Despite these criticisms, Gagnon (1975, 136) points out that there was much less of a shock reaction when *Human Sexual Response* was published as compared to the Kinsey reports. He believes this was for three main reasons. Firstly, Masters and Johnson's focus on anatomy and physiology meant their research was more removed from the main concerns of people's lives than the Kinsey team's research on human sexual behaviour. Secondly, the research by Kinsey and his colleagues created a more conducive environment for Masters and Johnson's project. It also gave people a discursive framework for better understanding sex researchers and their work. Thirdly, the legitimacy of Masters and Johnson's research was greatly enhanced by being 'performed under the umbrella of the medical and biological sciences' (Gagnon 1975, 136). Furthermore, when Masters and Johnson's work was criticised, the criticisms, on the whole were fairly restrained. Gagnon (1975, 137) argues there were essentially two main reasons for this. Firstly, many critics were aware that an overly critical reaction to Masters and Johnson's work might severely curtail opportunities for further sex research. This was generally seen as undesirable given the importance attached to Masters and Johnson's work. Secondly, one of the main reasons for Masters and Johnson's research was to develop effective therapies for people with sexual dysfunctions. Masters and Johnson strongly emphasised that sex is a natural response. In their view, sexual dysfunctions occur when this natural response is disrupted by anxieties and inhibitions. They believed that the role of sex therapy in these circumstances is to remove the impediments to natural sexual functioning. This way of framing their research and therapeutic agenda proved to be highly compatible with prevailing cultural beliefs that people's natural instincts, like their sexuality, should be liberated from the weight of unnecessary repression.

CONCLUSION

This chapter reviewed the nature and public impact of Masters and Johnson's (1966) research on human sexual response. It, firstly, examined the main reasons for the research, the location and funding of the research, and the main research questions which Masters and Johnson set out to answer. The chapter argued that while Masters and Johnson were not the first to directly study human sexual response, their approach was modelled on that of scientific medicine, and framed to address pressing public concerns about divorce and family break down in U.S. society. This helped to provide legitimacy for their project and further their research and therapeutic objectives.

After reviewing Masters' initial research with prostitutes, and highlighting its importance for his project, the chapter then examined the hiring of Virginia Johnson, and the recruitment of research participants for the next phase of the research. After orientating participants to the laboratory, Masters and Johnson observed, measured and recorded the physical sexual responses of 694 men and women over an eleven year period from 1954 to 1965. Their major finding was that male and female sexual response is so similar that it can be understood as occurring within a single human sexual response cycle. The chapter then outlined the four major stages of this cycle: excitement, plateau, orgasm and resolution.

Following this, the chapter then discussed the publication and reception of Masters and Johnson's (1966) famous book about their research, *Human Sexual Response*. Here, the chapter argued that there was a largely favourable reaction to their book. There was a general acceptance of its findings. The book was used to inaugurate courses on the physiology of human sexual response in numerous U.S. medical schools. The model of the human sexual response cycle was incorporated (in an amended form) into the *DSM-III* (1980) and subsequent editions of the *DSM* (American Psychiatric Association 1987; 1994; 2000), and many feminists lauded the work and emphasised its positive implications for women.

Finally, the chapter argued that when Masters and Johnson's (1966) research was criticised, the criticism focused much more on their research methods than their research findings. Their findings, including the centrepiece of their work — the human sexual response cycle — were, and largely still are, accepted as scientifically established facts. The following chapter, however, provides a critique of Masters and Johnson's model of the human sexual response cycle, and some of their claims about it.

5 A Critique of Masters and Johnson's Model of the Human Sexual Response Cycle

INTRODUCTION

In the previous chapter it was argued that Masters and Johnson's (1966) research attracted relatively little criticism. When it was criticised, it tended to be for their methods of investigation rather than their actual research findings. The findings themselves seem to have been generally accepted. The aim of this chapter, however, is to provide a critique of Masters and Johnson's main research findings expressed in their model of the four phase human sexual response cycle. It will be argued that a number of Masters and Johnson's claims, both about and within the model, are seriously defective and that many of these defects are best explained by taking into account the social context within which they worked. They will be criticised, in particular, for their claims about the originality of the four stage model of sexual response, the strongly essentialist basis of their response cycle, inconsistencies between their reported data and their model of the sexual response cycle, their ideological emphasis on the sexual similarities of males and females, and inaccurate research findings on human sexual response. The chapter begins, however, with a critical discussion of their claim that they were the first to construct a four phase model of human sexual response.

THE ORIGINALITY OF THE FOUR STAGE MODEL OF THE HUMAN SEXUAL RESPONSE CYCLE

Masters and Johnson's notion of a four stage human sexual response cycle is the centrepiece of their book *Human Sexual Response*. It apparently encapsulated the results of their laboratory sex research and helped to build their scientific reputations. It was, in effect, their answer to the question about what physical changes occur in males and females in response to effective sexual stimulation (Masters and Johnson 1966, 4). Masters, Johnson and Kolodny (1994, 41) claimed that Masters and Johnson 'were the first to devise a four-stage model to describe and explain ... natural physiological changes' in the body in response to effective sexual stimulation. This claim, however, is untrue. The Berlin neurologist, Albert Moll, had already divided the process of human sexual response into four stages in his book *The Sexual Life of the Child* published in 1912 (Money 1985, 177). According to Moll (1912, 26), 'In woman as in man, the curve of voluptuousness exhibits four phases.' What Masters and Johnson (1966) called excitement, plateau, orgasm and resolution, Moll (1912, 26) had previously termed 'an ascending limb, the equable voluptuous sensation, the acme, and the rapid decline.' Moreover, Moll's work was known to Masters and Johnson (1966, 329) as they cited it in *Human Sexual Response.*

When Masters and Johnson introduced the notion of a four phase sexual response cycle in the first chapter of *Human Sexual Response*, however, they gave no hint that Moll's previous conceptualisation might have influenced them in any way. On the contrary, they suggested that it was primarily their direct observations and physical measurements which enabled them to define and describe male and female sexual response cycles (Masters and Johnson 1966, 4). In a later work, Masters et al (1985, 78) confirmed that it was the findings of Masters and Johnson's earlier laboratory study (rather than any influence from Moll's work) which 'indicated that human sexual response could be described as a cycle with four stages....' How the results of their laboratory research square with their admission that they *arbitrarily* divided the sexual response cycle into four stages is not made clear (Masters and Johnson 1966, 4).

Human sexual response had also been divided into stages by the English physician Havelock Ellis. His theory of tumescence and detumescence was adopted from the work of Albert Moll (Ellis 1942, 20–7; Bullough 1994a, 83). This, too, was long before Masters and Johnson's (1966) research. Ellis (1936, 115) divided sexual response into two stages: 'tumescence,' where 'force is generated in the organism,' and 'detumescence' where 'that force is discharged during conjugation.' Ellis's discourse about the accumulation and discharge of force has clear parallels with Masters and Johnson's (1966, 6) description of 'maximum sexual tension' leading to orgasm and a 'period of tension loss' following orgasm. Robinson (1976, 126) has argued that, in many ways, Masters and Johnson's four stage cycle of sexual response is basically a refinement of Ellis's two stage model. Masters and Johnson's excitement and plateau stages, for example, correspond with Ellis's tumescence stage while the former's orgasm and resolution stages correspond with Ellis's detumescence stage.

Like Moll's (1912) work, Ellis's (1936) *Studies in the Psychology of Sex,* Volume Two, was known to Masters and Johnson (1966, 320) as they cited it in *Human Sexual Response.* If Masters and Johnson's notion of a four stage sexual response cycle was, in part, a refinement of Moll's and/or Ellis's models, and not acknowledged as such, then perhaps this was because Masters and Johnson felt under considerable pressure to produce original research findings. These findings were needed to help justify their controversial laboratory research and to protect their professional reputations and careers. Masters once stated, for example, that:

> If you do cancer research for ten years and don't come up with anything noteworthy, nobody is going to question you professionally. I went into sex research with the full knowledge that I had to win. I had to come up with something or I would have been destroyed professionally. (Belliveau and Richter 1971, 19–20)

THE ESSENTIALIST BASIS OF THE HUMAN SEXUAL RESPONSE CYCLE

At face value, the human sexual response cycle might appear to be the outcome of an empiricist approach to sex research where Masters and Johnson bracketed their preconceptions about sex and simply observed the 'facts' of human sexual response as it unfolded in the laboratory. A closer inspection, however, reveals that Masters and Johnson were influenced in their research by certain essentialist assumptions about sexuality. Like many other sex researchers, they seem to have believed that humans have a sexual drive which is inherent in human biology: 'The cycle of sexual response, with orgasm as the ultimate point in progression, generally is believed to develop from a drive of biologic-behavioral origin deeply integrated into the condition of human existence' (Masters and Johnson 1966, 127).

For Masters and Johnson, the human sex drive is basically a natural force inside individuals which is geared to the survival and reproduction of the human species. According to Johnson, the term 'sex drive' is scientifically imprecise but 'It's often used to mean the basic drive to reproduce' ('Playboy interview: Masters and Johnson' 1976, 150). Masters and Johnson rarely refer in an explicit way to the notion of a sex drive but it is clear from their work that they see normal sexual response as embodying psychological demands for copulation (implicitly stemming from the influence of an underlying sex drive) and a physical process designed to prepare the bodies of males and females for reproductive sex. The examples below indicate the ways in which Masters and Johnson interpret physiological changes in sexed bodies as being 'naturally' and exclusively geared to heterosexual copulation. 'Full penile erection is, for the male, obvious physiological evidence of a psychological demand for intromission. In exact parallel, full vaginal lubrication for the female is obvious physiological evidence of a psychological invitation for penetration' (Masters and Johnson 1970, 199). 'Just as penile erection is a direct physiologic expression of a psychologic demand to mount, so expansion and lubrication of the vaginal barrel provides direct physiologic indication of an obvious psychologic mounting invitation' (Masters and Johnson 1966, 68). Masters and Johnson (1966,

342), in turn, define the term 'mount' as meaning the onset of coitus when the penis is thrust into the vagina.

The concept of a sex drive in Masters and Johnson's account explains why people want to have sex and thereby set their sexual response cycles into motion. They want to have sex because they are born with an inner drive toward orgasm for the purpose of reproducing the species. Once the inborn sex drive builds to the point where it seeks release by causing a need for sexual stimulation, any stimulation encountered will set off the human sexual response cycle which follows the dictates of an 'inborn program, like the workings of a mechanical clock' (Tiefer 1995, 43). Once started, the cycle continues through an orderly sequence of events that tend to repeat themselves as long as effective sexual stimulation continues. This sequence of events prepares 'the bodies of two mates for reproductive union' (Kaplan 1978, 28). Heterosexual coitus seems to be pre-ordained by and emerges 'naturally' from the complementary psychological and physiological processes of males and females. As Boyle (1993, 78) puts it, Masters and Johnson's 'granting of volition to male and female genitals (erections which demanded intromission; vaginas which invited penetration) creates the impression that the only biologically correct way to deal with sexual excitement is to have heterosexual intercourse.'

As discussed in chapter 3, the essentialist basis of Masters and Johnson's model of the human sexual response cycle can be criticised on a number of grounds. Firstly, there is so far no conclusive evidence that human desire for sex is generated by a biological need. This notion of an innate human sex drive was criticised at least as far back as the 1950s when Masters and Johnson were first beginning their Sex Research Project. Beach (1956, 2–5), for example, pointed out that this notion was 'open to serious dispute' because it did not have anything to do with 'genuine biological or tissue needs.' He suggested that the concept of sex drive be replaced by that of 'sexual appetite' which is a 'product of experience' within a sociocultural context. Secondly, Masters and Johnson's (1966, 127) notion of an innate sex drive is posited without any specification of the means by which the alleged drive actually shapes human motivation and behaviour. The connection is just assumed. Finally, there is no evidence that an instinct or drive determines human sexual behaviour. The genetic determination of complex behaviour patterns only appears to exist in non-mammalian animal species (Laumann and Gagnon 1995, 185).

In the absence of a convincing account of an innate sex drive, Masters and Johnson's model of the human sexual response cycle faces two major problems. Firstly, the model is left without an adequate explanation of why people want to have sex in the first place so that they might set their sexual response cycles into motion. The model of the human sexual response cycle only describes what happens after sexual stimulation begins, not why it initially occurs.

Masters and Johnson have been criticised for ignoring the issue of sexual desire in their account of human sexual response, particularly since this might explain why a sexual response cycle is initially set in motion (Kaplan 1977; Lief 1977). The critics, however, have not always been sure why Masters and Johnson omitted a sexual desire stage from their model of the human sexual response cycle. Davison and Neale (1994, 366), for example, believe that Masters and Johnson omitted this stage from their model because they used sexually 'well-functioning volunteers' in their laboratory work, so the 'issue of desire or readiness to be sexual did not arise.' This explanation, however, seems doubtful for two main reasons. Firstly, Masters and Johnson (1966, 311) were aware of the importance of sexual motivation because they made a positive history of coital orgasm and masturbatory experience an explicit requirement for choosing their research participants. People with little or no sexual motivation would be much less likely to have the positive orgasmic history that Masters and Johnson required. Secondly, some of the research participants did occasionally 'fail' to sexually perform in the ways required by Masters and Johnson (1966, 312–14). Some of these 'failures' might well have been due, at least in part, to lack of adequate sexual motivation, and this is a possibility which Masters and Johnson (1966, 314) seem to acknowledge. In short, then, the issue of sexual desire or the 'readiness to be sexual' did arise in their research, and it would have been very surprising if it did not. It seems more likely that Masters and Johnson did not explicitly discuss sexual desire because, in their work, sexual desire is reduced to and explained in terms of a sex drive. This is not an unusual conflation as Gagnon and Parker (1995, 12) explain:

> Traditionally, sexual desire was assumed to be natural and automatic and heterosexual and universal. The penis desired the vagina and the vagina desired the penis.... Indeed, instead of desire, theorists wrote of lust, the drive or impulse which knew its own aims or goals.

Masters and Johnson (1966) could conceivably have discussed a stage of sexual motivation, (in terms of their concept of a sex drive), prior to the other stages of their model of the human sexual response cycle. However, their main research questions were not explicitly concerned with this issue. They were primarily concerned with what happens *after* effective sexual stimulation begins, and why men and women behave in the way they do when responding to this stimulation (Masters and Johnson 1966, 10). Consequently, their notion of a sex drive is barely mentioned in *Human Sexual Response*, and it exists mainly as an implicit underpinning of their model of sexual response. Masters and Johnson's omission of a concept of sexual desire ultimately led to a theoretical impasse in the understanding of human sexual response, and it was not until the mid-1970s that other sexologists began to discuss sexual desire as an integral part of the response process.

The second major problem stemming from the unsubstantiated sex drive underpinning of Masters and Johnson's human sexual response cycle is the difficulty of justifying their conviction that heterosexual coitus is the natural, universal and objective 'purpose' (and outcome) of human sexual response. Masters and Johnson's account gives the impression that the physiological processes which characterise human sexual response have their own intrinsic object or telos toward which they are inexorably moving, namely, coital sex for the purpose of reproducing new members of the species. According to Margolis (1987, 147), however, what is 'typically required for the survival and reproduction of the *species* is quite compatible with a variety of sexual behavior patterns — and ... a variety of reproductive capacity (even the distributed absence of such capacity) — with respect to individual organisms.'

This means that not only may individuals be infertile, they may be voluntarily childless, sexually abstinent, or engage in non-reproductive sexual activity without homo sapiens as a species necessarily failing to adequately reproduce. It is conceivable that only a small proportion of all sexual activity devoted to biological reproduction would be sufficient to maintain the survival of the species (Warren 1986, 145).

Sociological, historical and anthropological documentation of the enormous diversity of human sexual practices between and within societies presents a major obstacle to the assumption of an inexorable 'coital imperative' because it indicates that a great variety of sexual activities are compatible with the physiological processes of the human body (Laumann et al 1994; Tannahill 1989; Gregersen 1994). Masters and Johnson's strongly essentialist view of sexuality has trouble explaining sexual diversity because it assumes the existence of an innate sex drive which knows 'its own aims or goals' and which expresses itself in terms of psychological demands and physiological preparation for heterosexual coitus. Masters and Johnson do not explain how coitus could represent a natural, universal and self-evident standard of normal sexual functioning but they have interpreted their observations of human sexual physiology as if it was, and then tried to claim back these same observations as proof they had found a correct and objective standard.

INCONSISTENCIES BETWEEN MASTERS AND JOHNSON'S DATA AND THEIR MODEL OF THE HUMAN SEXUAL RESPONSE CYCLE

Masters and Johnson (1966) claimed that their model of the human sexual response cycle was constructed on the basis of the research data which they gathered in their laboratory study and reported in *Human Sexual Response*. Their model of human sexual response, however, can be further criticised because in certain important ways it seems to be inconsistent with their own reported findings.

Firstly, Masters and Johnson (1966) claim that human sexual response occurs in a symmetrical cycle for both males and females. They state that an individual's progression from orgasm to resolution is an exact reversal of the previous progression from excitement to plateau.

> The human male and female resolve from the height of their orgasmic expressions into the last or resolution phase of the sexual cycle. This involutionary period of tension loss develops as a *reverse reaction pattern* that returns the individual through plateau and excitement levels to an unstimulated state. (Masters and Johnson 1966, 6; emphasis added)

Masters and Johnson (1966) point out that in the resolution stage males enter a unique refractory period while females do not. Yet they apparently do not recognise the consequences of this important male/female difference for their conception of sexual response as a cycle. Robinson (1976, 127) points out that if human sexual response really occurred in a symmetrical cycle then males would also have to enter a refractory period just prior to orgasm. Masters and Johnson (1966), of course, found no evidence of such a refractory period and so their claim of a symmetrical cycle for male sexual response is unsubstantiated. Their concept of cyclical sexual response, however, has more plausibility in the case of females who do not experience a refractory period and have at least the potential of being re-stimulated to further orgasms.

Secondly, there is the question of how appropriate it is to divide the process of human sexual response into four stages, each corresponding to a discrete set of physiological events. Masters and Johnson's four stage model of sexual response is based on the implicit assumption that the events of sexual physiology occur in a series of discrete stages rather than in a continuous process. This is contrary to the findings of their own research and their admission that sexual responses, such as penile erection and vaginal lubrication, continue through more than one stage (Masters and Johnson 1966, 7). The actual continuity of physiological processes is further underlined by the fact that the individuals experiencing effective sexual stimulation do not suddenly jump 'from one stage to the next' as they respond (Mahoney 1983, 123). Masters and Johnson (1966, 4) admit that their four part division of the human sexual response cycle is arbitrary but they claim it helps to describe certain fleeting physiological variations of sexual response which may only appear in one stage of the cycle. The disadvantage of the model, however, is that it seems to misrepresent the unfolding of physiological processes which it is meant to illuminate.

Thirdly, there is the problem of how Masters and Johnson can justify the demarcation of the excitement stage from the plateau stage in their model of sexual response (Robinson 1976, 127). Masters and Johnson admit, for example, that the stages cannot always be clearly distinguished from one another and they themselves show some confusion over how to demarcate them (Masters et al 1985, 78). At times they have suggested that males and females can still be in the excitement stage long after they have achieved full erection or lubrication; at other times they have claimed that males and females could reach the plateau stage even without full erection or lubrication (Robinson 1976, 127).

Robinson (1976, 130) has argued that, in relation to males, there does not seem to be any justification for making a distinction between the excitement and plateau stages of sexual response. None of the physiological processes described by Masters and Johnson are confined to only one of these two stages in a way that would make that stage distinctive. Instead, there is a continuity of physiological processes through these two stages. Robinson (1976, 129) illustrates this by pointing to inconsistencies in Masters and Johnson's account of the sexual response pattern of the testes. On the one hand, Masters and Johnson (1966, 206) state (in line with their stage model) that the 'testes evidence specific reaction patterns during each of the four phases of the sexual response cycle'; yet, on the other hand, their own account of how the testes respond to sexual stimulation indicates that the testes continually elevate through the excitement and plateau stages until they are positioned against the perineum, just prior to orgasm and ejaculation (Masters and Johnson 1966, 206–7).

The four stage model is also unable to cope very well with the brief physiological events which typically occur in males just prior to orgasm, such as the emergence of pre-ejaculatory fluid from the penis (Robinson 1976, 129). Masters and Johnson try to accommodate these pre-orgasmic events within their model by basically creating stages within the plateau stage. To do this they are drawn into using such expressions as 'advanced plateau', 'late in the plateau phase', and 'terminal plateau phase' (Robinson 1976, 130). Their delineation of stages within the plateau stage makes their choice of the term 'plateau' an incongruous one and, taken together, these problems indicate serious deficiencies in their model of male sexual response. Robinson (1976, 130) concludes that:

> As far as the male is concerned...the scheme of four phases proves altogether irrelevant. It merely creates the impression of scientific precision where none exists. Ironically, Havelock Ellis's doctrine of tumescence and detumescence, though more general, turns out to be a more appropriate and far less pretentious abstraction, since it allows for both those phenomena that are cumulative and those that are sudden and evanescent rather than imposing boxlike categories that correspond to neither.

Masters and Johnson's four stage model of sexual response has similar problems in relation to females. Female sexual response is also characterised by physiological continuities, such as the development of the sex flush on the body, and by brief physiological events which typically occur just prior to orgasm, such as the vivid colour changes of the labia minora. The discrete stages of the model again have difficulty capturing physiological changes which are not distinctive to one stage or which occur just prior to orgasm. In the latter case, Masters and Johnson again try to delineate stages within the plateau stage in order to fit these pre-orgasmic events into their model (Robinson 1976, 131).

Masters and Johnson's distinction between excitement and plateau stages of sexual response seems to derive its justification with reference to female sexual response. In females, Masters and Johnson found there were distinct physiological changes which could be taken as representing an intermediate stage between excitement and orgasm. These changes included the cessation of vaginal lubrication; the withdrawal of the clitoris into its hood; and the phenomenon of the orgasmic platform where the outer one-third of the vagina swells with blood and greatly reduces the size of the vaginal opening. Robinson (1976, 131–2) argues that Masters and Johnson's model was primarily constructed to highlight the female orgasmic platform in order to debunk the Freudian distinction between vaginal and clitoral orgasms. Masters and Johnson's (1966) position was that female orgasms involve the same physiological responses regardless of the method or site of sexual stimulation. A key physiological response is the development of the orgasmic platform (which, for Masters and Johnson, represented the start of the plateau stage) and 'its pleasurable resolution in contractions' (which marked the end of that stage) (Robinson 1976, 132).

> Precisely, however, because the orgasmic platform is the centrepiece of their case against the Freudians, Masters and Johnson have allowed it, perhaps unwittingly, to dictate the conceptual scheme with which they seek to comprehend all other sexual processes as well. And although that scheme succeeds admirably in bringing the orgasmic platform to the focus of attention, it is largely meaningless as a general description of human sexual response. It thus contributes greatly to the sense of intellectual confusion and ungainliness that characterises their work as a whole. (Robinson 1976, 133)

It should be noted that Masters and Johnson were either unaware of, or chose to disregard, Robinson's (1976) detailed criticisms of their four stage model of sexual response. In later publications, for example, Masters, Johnson and Kolodny (1985; 1994) presented the original model without any reference to Robinson's criticisms and maintained that the notion of a plateau stage of sexual response is equally applicable to males and females. By contrast, the *DSM-III* (1980) omitted the plateau stage altogether from its model of sexual response, and this omission was repeated in the *DSM-IIIR* (1987), the *DSM-IV* (1994), and the *DSM-IV-TR* (2000).

THE IDEOLOGICAL EMPHASIS ON SEXUAL SIMILARITY

The notion of a single human sexual response cycle allowed Masters and Johnson to highlight the essential similarity of male and female sexual response by locating each of these responses within a common model. In their book *Human Sexual Response*, they also emphasised that their discovery of sexual similarity was a major finding of their research:

> again and again attention will be drawn to direct parallels in human sexual response that exist to a degree never previously appreciated. Attempts to answer the challenge inherent in the question, 'What do men and women do in response to effective sexual stimulation?' have emphasized the *similarities, not the differences*, in the anatomy and physiology of human sexual response. (Masters and Johnson 1966, 8; emphasis in original)

Masters and Johnson (1966) did find many similarities in the sexual responses of males and females. For example, both males and females generally experience myotonia, vasocongestion, increased heart rate and blood pressure during sexual response. Similarly, during orgasm, the muscular contractions of the vagina, penis and anuses of both sexes occur at 0.8 second intervals. On the other hand, Masters and Johnson's research also indicated there were some significant differences between male and female sexual response. They state, for example, that:

> Only one sexual response pattern has been diagrammed for the human male...[and variations in response have more to do with its duration than intensity]. Comparably, three different sexual response patterns have been diagrammed for the human female.... There is great variation in both the intensity and duration of female orgasmic experience, while the male tends to follow standard patterns of ejaculatory reaction with less individual variation. (Masters and Johnson 1966, 4–6)

Masters and Johnson (1966) found that males typically move from the excitement stage through plateau to orgasm and then experience a refractory period during which they cannot be restimulated to orgasm. This refractory period may lead either to complete resolution or to effective restimulation once the refractory period is over. By contrast, Masters and Johnson found that females have three possible patterns of sexual response. Firstly, females can have a pattern similar to males where they move from excitement through plateau to orgasm and resolution, even though they do not experience a refractory period. Secondly, females have the potential of returning to orgasm from anywhere within the resolution stage if effective sexual stimulation is recommenced (Masters and Johnson 1966, 6–7). This means that women have a capacity to experience multiple orgasms which men do not have. Thirdly, some women have the ability to maintain an orgasmic experience for a fairly long period of time. Masters and Johnson (1966, 131) regard this as a 'rare reaction' which they call 'status orgasmus'. They explain it as follows:

> This physiological state of stress is created either by a series of rapidly recurrent orgasmic experiences between which no recordable plateau-phase intervals can be demonstrated, or by a single, long-continued orgasmic episode. Subjective report, together with visual impression of involuntary variation in peripheral myotonia, suggests that the woman actually is ranging with extreme rapidity between successive orgasmic peaks and a baseline of advanced plateau-phase tension. Status orgasmus may last from 20 to more than 60 seconds.... (Masters and Johnson 1966, 131)

A further important difference which Masters and Johnson (1966) found between male and female sexual response is that only males ejaculate while females do not.

Given that Masters and Johnson's (1966) own research findings point to some significant differences between male and female sexual response, whey then did they insist on only highlighting the similarities? In Irvine's (1990b, 17) view, their decision was ideological rather than scientific. She argues that Masters and Johnson selectively highlighted their findings on similarity to address public fears and concerns about important social changes in U.S. society. By the early 1960s, the divorce rate had begun to increase, the 'age of marriage rose and the birthrate dropped' (Irvine 1990b, 18). These developments led to publicly expressed anxieties about gender roles, sexuality, marriage and the family. Masters and Johnson (1970, 369) themselves believed that half the marriages in the United States were sexually dysfunctional and that sexual dysfunction was the biggest single cause of divorce and family break down (Masters and Johnson 1966, vi). They positioned their research on sexual response, from the very beginning, as an attempt to scientifically solve the problem of sexual dysfunction and its perceived threat to marriage and the family.

Irvine (1990b) argues that Masters and Johnson emphasised the sexual similarities of males and females because they saw similarity as a basis for equality in the bedroom, mutual understanding, and more harmonious marital relationships. They assumed that once males and females realised how sexually similar they are to each other, their mutual enjoyment of sex would improve, their relationships would strengthen and the threat of sexual dysfunction to marriage and the family would subside (Segal 1994, 94).

Masters and Johnson's (1966) emphasis on sexual similarity was positive for women in some ways because it broke with the dominant nineteenth century emphasis on the 'natural' *differences* between the sexes in which women were not only considered to be different to men but also unequal. The stress on sexual similarity challenged the idea that women were sexually inferior to men. Feminists were able to use these findings to challenge the sexual double-standard and restrictions on women's sexual autonomy. On the other hand, Masters and Johnson's stress on sexual similarity was always going to be limited as a means of addressing gender inequality. Their ideas were advanced 'in the absence of any broader critique of male dominance and of heterosexism', and they assumed that scientific proof of sexual similarity was more important for social change than political struggle. It seems extremely unlikely that gender equality will ever be achieved simply by a common recognition that men's and women's bodies sexually respond in similar ways (Irvine 1990b, 20–2).

INACCURATE RESEARCH FINDINGS

In *Human Sexual Response*, Masters and Johnson assumed that their research sample was large enough and sufficiently varied to give them a comprehensive and accurate picture of human sexual response. They assumed that the physiological data they gathered from their small non-representative sample could be taken as representative of the sexual responses of all human beings. This assumption was reflected in, among other things, the title of their work, *Human Sexual Response*, which implies that their research data is representative of humans *as such*. This was an unfortunate assumption because it now appears that two of their key findings on 'human sexual response' are wrong. These findings concern male multiple orgasm and female ejaculation.

Masters and Johnson's (1966) view was that males are not capable of multiple orgasm. They reported that one of the major differences between male and female sexual response is that males experience a refractory period after orgasm while females do not. During this period, males are not capable of being restimulated to higher levels of sexual tension or orgasm. They argued that females, on the other hand, do not experience a refractory period and so are physiologically capable of experiencing multiple orgasms.

> The male has a unique refractory period which develops as the last, irregular, nonexpulsive contractions of the penile urethra occur and is maintained until sexual tension in the male has been reduced to low excitement-phase levels of response. The female has no such refractory reaction. She generally maintains higher levels of stimulative susceptibility during the immediate postorgasmic period. She usually is capable of return to repeated orgasmic experience without postorgasmic loss of sexual tension below plateau-phase levels of response. (Masters and Johnson 1966, 283–4; emphasis added)

Subsequent research, however, has refuted Masters and Johnson's (1966) view that male multiple orgasm is not possible. Robbins and Jensen (1978) studied thirteen men aged from 22 to 56 years who said that they experienced multiple orgasms prior to ejaculating.

> The men reported from 3 to 10 orgasms per lovemaking session (prior to ejaculation) and, while their responsiveness appeared to have something to do with the mood and circumstances of the sexual encounter, they found their multiple orgasmic response to be fairly reliable experiencing it in approximately 4 out of 5 intercourse experiences. Under optimal conditions when his partner was cooperative, one male experienced as many as 30 orgasms in one session of sexual intercourse lasting approximately 1 hour. (Robbins and Jensen 1978, 23)

Robbins and Jensen (1978) were able to confirm the existence of male multiple orgasm by taking physiological measurements of the sexual responses of a male research participant in their laboratory. This man experienced three separate orgasms within a matter of seconds. His final orgasm coincided with ejaculation.

Hartman and Fithian (1985) have also confirmed the existence of male multiple orgasm through their laboratory investigation of male sexual response. They used a nine-channel recorder to monitor men's sexual responses during masturbation and coitus. They found that of 282 male research participants they studied, 33 were capable of multiple orgasms. The number of orgasms experienced by these men during the research ranged from two to sixteen, with an average of four. Hartman and Fithian (1985) reported that their physiological measurements of male multiple orgasms were very similar to those of female multiple orgasms. 'In fact, unless we looked at the name of the subject, we could not tell whether a chart we studied was that of a female or male multi-orgasmic response' (Hartman and Fithian 1985, 2).

Masters and Johnson responded with contradictory statements when confronted with research findings which refuted their own. On the one hand, they held to their original view that men 'are not able to have multiple orgasm if it is defined in the same way' as for females (Masters et al 1985, 92). Yet, on the other hand, and in the same paragraph, they contradicted themselves by admitting that 'it does appear that at least a few men have the capacity to have multiple orgasms before a true refractory period sets in....' (Masters et al 1985, 92).

If Masters and his colleagues (1985) were now prepared to admit, at least on some level, that male multiple orgasm does exist, then how did they miss it in their 'ground breaking' laboratory research?

Hartman and Fithian (1985, 151) learned from their personal correspondence with Masters and Johnson that the latter did not know anything about male multiple orgasm and had never researched the topic. Because they did not know anything about it, they did not actively look for evidence of it in their research. That is, their lack of knowledge of the topic, and their preconceptions, affected the planning and conduct of their research. This would have meant, for example, that Masters and Johnson did not try to recruit male volunteers with this capacity, or that if they did unwittingly recruit them, Masters and Johnson did not raise the subject with them or ask them to demonstrate this capacity in the laboratory. When Masters and Johnson did not look for evidence, and did not find it, their preconceptions would have been undisturbed. They apparently took the absence of evidence of multiple orgasms by their male research participants to be evidence of the absence of a capacity for multiple orgasm in the 'human male.'

In addition, it now seems clear that Masters and Johnson's (1966) original research confused two separate physiological processes in males — orgasm and ejaculation — and assumed they were the same process. Throughout *Human Sexual Response,* and particularly in their chapter on 'The Male Orgasm (Ejaculation),' it is evident that Masters and Johnson saw male 'orgasm' and 'ejaculation' as synonymous terms for a single physiological process. Because of this confusion, they believed that a refractory period *had* to develop after every male orgasm/ejaculation and that this naturally prevents males from experiencing multiple orgasms.

The problem with Masters and Johnson's (1966) view is that orgasm and ejaculation are separate physiological processes. They usually occur together but they can occur independently of each other. Kinsey et al (1948, 158–9), for example, pointed out that in pre-adolescent males, orgasm without ejaculation is the rule, and even in some adult males 'who deliberately constrict their genital muscles' orgasm occurs without ejaculation. Ejaculation is also known to occur without orgasm, such as when erectile centres in the spinal cord are given electrical stimulation (Kinsey et al 1948, 159). In their later work, Masters and Johnson acknowledged that 'Male orgasm and ejaculation are not one and the same process' (Masters et al 1985, 90). By doing so, they conceded that their original research 'finding' on this was mistaken.

The distinction between orgasm and ejaculation is important for understanding male multiple orgasm. The research on men who are capable of experiencing multiple orgasms suggests that these men have learned to distinguish the orgasm response from the ejaculatory response. They can apparently inhibit the ejaculatory response so that they can have a number of orgasms without ejaculating (Robbins and Jensen 1978; Hartman and Fithian 1985; Dunn and Trost 1989). This means that a refractory period does not automatically follow male orgasm, as Masters and Johnson (1966) believed, otherwise male multiple orgasm would be impossible. It seems more likely that the refractory period occurs after *ejaculation* and represents the time taken before another orgasm and/or ejaculation is possible (Mahoney 1983, 133).

Masters and Johnson (1966) also denied the existence of female ejaculation. In this case, they were aware of reports about it but they gave them no credence. Because of this they did not seriously investigate the possibility of female ejaculation in their laboratory research even though their primary aim was to find out what happens to men and women as they respond to effective sexual stimulation. Even when some of their female research participants reported a sensation of ejaculating fluid during orgasm, Masters and Johnson dismissed their reports. They did this on the basis that they believed female ejaculation to be an artefact of male interpretations of women's experiences. They believed that these interpretations had possibly misled their research participants.

> During the first stage of subjective progression in orgasm, the sensation of intense clitoral-pelvic awareness has been described by a number of women as occurring concomitantly with a sense of bearing down or expelling. Often a feeling of receptive opening was expressed. This last sensation was reported only by parous study subjects, a small number of whom expressed some concept of having an actual fluid emission or of expending in some concrete fashion. Previous male interpretation of these subjective reports may have resulted in the erroneous but widespread concept that female ejaculation is an integral part of female orgasmic expression. (Masters and Johnson 1966, 135)

Reports of female ejaculation, however, are not confined to Masters and Johnson's (1966) research. They span many centuries and come from a number of different societies (Sevely 1987, Ch.3). Scientific interest in the topic was rekindled by Sevely and Bennett (1978) who criticised Masters and Johnson's (1966) decision not to investigate it. Sevely and Bennett (1978) concluded from their research that it is possible for women to ejaculate. They argued that, anatomically, women have tissues surrounding their urethras which are homologous to the male prostate and develop embryologically from the same source. In males, the prostate secretes a liquid which comprises a large proportion of the male ejaculate. Similarly in women, Sevely and Bennett (1978) argued that the 'female prostate' may be capable of ejaculating fluid from the urethra. They called for empirical research to establish whether or not women actually did ejaculate and referred to anecdotal evidence from both females and males on the occurrence of female ejaculation.

Subsequent research has demonstrated that Sevely and Bennett (1978) were right and that many women do, in fact, expel fluid from the urethra during orgasm. In some women this fluid is chemically different from urine. The phenomenon has been observed and filmed and is now accepted by almost all researchers (Darling et al 1990, 32–3; Irvine 1990a, 166; Bullough 1994a, 254). Even the previously sceptical Masters and Johnson admitted that they themselves have 'observed several cases of women who expelled a type of fluid that was not urine' (Masters et al 1985, 88). Research is continuing into this phenomenon and questions still remain about the source of the fluid, its actual composition and the number of women who are capable of ejaculating (Bullough 1994a, 254; Masters et al 1985, 88). Sevely and Bennett, (1978, 18–19) argued that Masters and Johnson's (1966) failure to investigate female ejaculation, even though they were prompted by cues about its possible occurrence, is best explained by their adherence to a dominant paradigm on female sexuality in which females were held not to ejaculate. Allegiance to this paradigm blinded them to the existence of evidence which did not fit prevailing scientific beliefs.

In short, Masters and Johnson's (1966) denial of the existence of male multiple orgasm and female ejaculation is an ironic one given that their research emphasised the similarities rather than the differences in male and female sexual response. Masters and Johnson 'found' that two of the main sex differences in 'human sexual response' are that only females are capable of multiple orgasm and that only males can ejaculate. They played down these 'differences', however, and highlighted the sexual similarities of men and women for ideological reasons. Yet, at the same time, they were unaware of the way in which their own preconceptions and prejudices had helped to establish the 'factuality' of these key sex 'differences' in the first place.

CONCLUSION

This chapter provided a critique of Masters and Johnson's (1966) model of the human sexual response cycle: the centrepiece of their research on human sexual response. Firstly, the chapter argued that, contrary to Masters and Johnson's claims, they were not the first to develop a four stage model of human sexual response. The Berlin neurologist, Albert Moll, had developed such a model in his book *The Sexual Life of the Child*, published in 1912. The English physician, Havelock Ellis, had also developed a two stage model of sexual response prior to Masters and Johnson. Masters and Johnson were aware of this earlier work but they did not acknowledge that it had influenced them in the development of their own model. Instead, they claimed that their model was derived from their laboratory research. I argued that if Masters and Johnson's model of a four stage sexual response cycle was influenced by the earlier work of Moll and/or Ellis, and not acknowledged, then it may have been because Masters and Johnson felt under considerable pressure to produce new and original research findings to justify their controversial laboratory research.

Secondly, the chapter identified and criticised certain essentialist assumptions underpinning Masters and Johnson's model of the human sexual response cycle. The chapter argued that Masters and Johnson failed to provide a convincing account of the existence of a biological sex drive in humans, and that their model of the human sexual response cycle was unable to explain *why* people want to have sex or *why* the sexual responses of males and females are naturally and exclusively geared to heterosexual coitus.

Thirdly, the chapter examined the relationship between Masters and Johnson's reported findings on human sexual response and their model of the human sexual response cycle. The chapter argued that there was a series of inconsistencies between their findings and the model even though Masters and Johnson claimed that the model was constructed on the basis of the findings reported in *Human Sexual Response*.

Fourthly, the chapter discussed how Masters and Johnson emphasised the sexual similarities between males and females even though they 'found' both similarities and differences in their research. It was argued that this was done for ideological rather than scientific reasons. Masters and Johnson were attempting to address important public concerns about gender relations, sexuality, marriage and the family. They believed that if males and females were aware of how sexually similar they are, then this would lead to fewer sexual dysfunctions, better sex lives, improved marriages and fewer divorces and family break-ups.

Finally, the chapter examined how and why Masters and Johnson made inaccurate research findings concerning male multiple orgasm and female ejaculation. I argued that Masters and Johnson did not know about male multiple orgasm, did not research the topic, and falsely generalised their 'findings' from a small unrepresentative sample of men to the 'human male'. They also conflated orgasm and ejaculation which are two separate physiological processes in males. In the case of female ejaculation, I argued that Masters and Johnson dismissed reports of this phenomenon from some of their female research participants because they were sure it did not occur and that the women were misinterpreting their own experiences. In the light of these arguments, it seems ironic that males and females may be more sexually similar, in physiological terms, than even Masters and Johnson realised, and that two of the major differences they 'found' — that males are not capable of multiple orgasm, and that females do not ejaculate — were largely constructed out of their own preconceptions and prejudices.

However, despite the various problems with Masters and Johnson's model of the human sexual response cycle, it was not just a way of encapsulating their 'scientific' findings on human sexual response. It also played a key role in the development of their sex therapy program. It was used to provide clinical norms of healthy sexual functioning from which sexual dysfunctions could be distinguished. The following chapter takes up this issue and provides a critique of Masters and Johnson's concept and classification of sexual dysfunction.

6 A Critique of Masters and Johnson's Concept and Classification of Sexual Dysfunction

INTRODUCTION

The concept of sexual dysfunction is central to the theory and practice of sex therapy. It is defined in relation to 'healthy' or 'normal' sexual functioning and refers to sexual 'problems' which are diagnosed and treated by sex therapists. Masters and Johnson developed clinical norms of sexual functioning based on their model of the human sexual response cycle and the ability of men and women to 'satisfactorily' engage in heterosexual coitus. Their concept and classification of sexual dysfunction was developed in relation to these norms. In the specialist and popular literature on human sexuality this concept and system of classification are often presented with little criticism probably because they are believed to be based on objective scientific data (see, for example, Masters and Johnson 1970; Kaplan 1978; Masters et al 1985; Pertot 1985; Llewellyn-Jones 1986 and 1987; Reinisch with Beasley 1991; Masters et al 1994; Kolodny 2001).

This chapter will argue that Masters and Johnson's (1970) concept and classification of sexual dysfunction are not simply based on objective discoveries by value free scientists but that they have been implicitly constructed with reference to dominant Western beliefs and values about sexuality. In particular, it will be argued that Masters and Johnson's work represents the medicalisation of 'deviant' sexual response and rests on questionable essentialist, heterosexist and gender biased views of sexuality.

The chapter will begin by discussing Masters and Johnson's standard of healthy sexual functioning and their concept of sexual dysfunction. This will be followed by an outline of their sexual dysfunction nosology. The remainder of the chapter will critically discuss the major flaws in this nosology and later versions of it. In particular, the nosology will be criticised for its reliance on a model of sexual functioning which has limited generalisability as a set of clinical norms; its numerous gender biases in the classification of sexual dysfunction; its hetero-coital bias; its omission of issues of sexual desire; its medicalisation of deviant sexual response; and its overconfident assumption that sexual dysfunctions are sexual problems and vice versa.

SEXUAL HEALTH AND SEXUAL DYSFUNCTION

Despite the problems with Masters and Johnson's (1966) findings on sexual physiology, their model of the human sexual response cycle was nevertheless used in their second book *Human Sexual Inadequacy* (1970) as a main reference point for studying 'deviant' sexual response. Their approach was explicitly modelled on that of scientific medicine. 'It is noteworthy that all of medical science is based on understanding normal anatomy and physiology before meaningful advances can be made in treating abnormalities' (Masters et al 1985, 21).

Masters and Johnson (1970) regarded their model of the human sexual response cycle as providing a standard of healthy sexual functioning. Their view of health seems to have been influenced by the 'biomedical model' which provides the conceptual underpinnings of modern scientific medicine (Capra 1983, 118). In the biomedical model, the human body is viewed as a machine, and the health of the body is believed to depend on the smooth mechanical functioning of its parts. Masters and Johnson, too, seem to regard the human body as a machine. They conceptualise human sexual response in terms of a clockwork model which progresses through its pre-set stages as long as it is powered by effective sexual stimulation. In the biomedical model, disease is viewed as a breakdown in the mechanical functioning of the body. Likewise, Masters and Johnson regard sexual dysfunction as a breakdown in the clockwork model of human sexual response. The machine is stimulated but its parts will not erect, lubricate, make contractions or ejaculate. The parts are apparently not functioning as they 'should,' as nature or evolution intended (Tiefer 1988, 19).

The term 'sexual dysfunction' seems appropriate to refer to mechanical breakdown. The prefix 'dys' means bad, ill, painful or disordered while the term 'function' means something that acts or operates in a certain way or according to a particular purpose (Lazarus 1989, 90). The combined form of these terms, 'dysfunction', thus means an act or operation which is abnormal, painful or impaired. The very use of the term 'dysfunction' biases thinking about sexual problems from the outset toward a physical and performance oriented conceptualisation (Mahoney 1983, 557). This can be seen very clearly in Masters and Johnson's own work. In *Human Sexual Response*, for example, they defined sexual inadequacy as 'Any degree of sexual response that is not sufficient for the isolated demand of the moment; may be constant or transitory *inability of performance*' (Masters and Johnson 1966, 344; emphasis added). It can also be seen in their later work where Masters et al (1985, 495) define sexual dysfunctions as 'conditions in which the ordinary *physical responses* of sexual function are impaired' (emphasis added).

Masters and Johnson (1970) were not content, however, to just produce a general definition of sexual dysfunction. In *Human Sexual Inadequacy* they also produced what is probably the first new system for classifying 'sexual dysfunctions' since the Middle Ages (Boyle 1994, 108). Their new system replaced an earlier classification of 'sexual dysfunctions' into 'impotence' and 'frigidity' (Boyle 1994, 104). Masters and Johnson's system of classification is described below.

MASTERS AND JOHNSON'S (1970) NOSOLOGY OF SEXUAL DYSFUNCTION

In their nosology, Masters and Johnson identified four main types of male sexual dysfunction:

1. 'Premature ejaculation': this occurs when a man is unable to delay his ejaculation for a sufficient period of time during penis in vagina intercourse so that his partner is satisfied (orgasms) in at least half of their coital encounters (Masters and Johnson 1970, 92).
2. 'Ejaculatory Incompetence': this arises when a man is unable to ejaculate in his partner's vagina (Masters and Johnson 1970, 116). The dysfunction may be primary (lifelong) or secondary (have developed after at least one successful performance).
3. 'Primary Impotence': this refers to a man's lifelong inability to develop or maintain an erection sufficient to permit coitus. 'Secondary Impotence' is when a man has produced an erection sufficient to accomplish at least one successful coital encounter but who otherwise has difficulty achieving or sustaining an erection (Masters and Johnson 1970, 157).
4. 'Dyspareunia': this means painful or difficult coitus (Masters and Johnson 1970, 266).

Masters and Johnson also identified three main types of female sexual dysfunction:

1. a) 'Primary Orgasmic Dysfunction': this refers to a woman's lifelong inability to achieve orgasm from all forms of attempted physical stimulation (Masters and Johnson 1970, 227).
   b) 'Situational Orgasmic Dysfunction': this is when a woman has had an orgasm on at least one occasion but who otherwise has difficulties reaching orgasm. There are three sub-categories of situational orgasmic dysfunction:
      i) 'Masturbatory Orgasmic Inadequacy': this occurs when a woman has been unable to achieve an orgasm via masturbation by herself or a partner but she can reach orgasm during coitus.
      ii) 'Coital Orgasmic Inadequacy': this refers to a woman who has never been able to achieve an orgasm during coitus but who

has been able to reach orgasm through other means such as masturbation or oral-genital contact.

iii) 'Random Orgasmic Inadequacy': this refers to a woman who has been able to reach orgasm at least once from both manipulation and coitus but who is rarely orgasmic and usually feels minimal or no physical need for sexual activity (Masters and Johnson 1970, 240). Masters and Johnson (1970, 247) further suggest, from one of their case histories of a woman with 'random orgasmic inadequacy', that 'low sexual tension' is also a potential clinical entity.

2. 'Vaginismus': this refers to an intense involuntary muscle spasm of the vaginal introitus (entrance of the vagina) that impedes or prevents penile penetration (Masters and Johnson 1970, 250). Vaginismus may be primary or secondary.

3. 'Dyspareunia': this again means painful or difficult coitus (Masters and Johnson 1970, 266).

Masters and Johnson's (1970) new system for classifying sexual dysfunctions was generally regarded as an advance and improvement on the earlier classification of dysfunctions into 'impotence' and 'frigidity.' The earlier terms were criticised for two main reasons. Firstly, they were diagnostically imprecise. Faulk (1973, 258) points out, for example, that 'frigidity' was used as a blanket term to cover a variety of different female conditions including lack of interest in sex, failure to become sexually aroused, failure to find sex pleasurable, difficulty or failure in reaching orgasm, failure to achieve coital orgasm and vaginismus. Similarly, 'impotence' could denote a variety of male conditions including low sexual desire, difficulties in obtaining or maintaining an erection, premature ejaculation, and ejaculatory incompetence (Rosen 1983, 81; Rosen 1996, 499). Secondly, the terms 'impotence' and 'frigidity' are pejorative and may stigmatise patients. The term 'frigidity,' for example, may suggest that patients with this diagnosis are emotionally cold, unfeeling and indifferent while patients diagnosed with 'impotence' may be seen as weak, ineffectual and powerless (Elliott 1985, 51).

Masters and Johnson's (1970) new nosology seemed to be a scientific advance over the old one, not only because it relied on their research on human sexual response but because it avoided some of the pitfalls of the old system of classification. Masters and Johnson (1970), for example, did not use the term 'frigidity' in their work, and so they avoided both the problems with its diagnostic imprecision and its pejorative overtones. Curiously, though, they did retain the term 'impotence'. They avoided any imprecision by defining it as erectile dysfunction and they carefully distinguished it from premature ejaculation and ejaculatory incompetence. However, they do not seem to have considered, or to have been concerned about, the way in which patients might find 'impotence' to be a 'stigmatizing and stress-inducing' label (Rosen and Leiblum 1992, 8). The same might be said about other diagnostic categories like 'ejaculatory incompetence' or 'premature ejaculation'.

'Within the field of sexology since 1970, Masters and Johnson's' nosology 'has served as the prototype for the diagnosis...of sexual dysfunctions' (Irvine 1990a, 192). Their categories were adopted by the *DSM-III* (1980) 'and are now considered official "mental disorders"' (Irvine 1990a, 193). Masters, Johnson and Kolodny (1985; 1994) have continued to reproduce their nosology in subsequent works with little criticism or amendment. The following section discusses some of the major problems with their nosology.

THE NOSOLOGY IS BASED ON A MODEL OF NORMAL SEXUAL RESPONSE WHICH HAS LIMITED GENERALISABILITY

Tiefer (1992, 233) has argued that the 'critique of current sexual dysfunction nosology must begin with an analysis of the appropriateness of basing clinical sexuality norms on 'the human sexual response cycle' as proposed by Masters and Johnson....' She has extensively criticised the generalisability of their research findings on human sexual response. Some of her criticisms were previously made by Singer (1973) but her critique (1992) forms the basis of the discussion in this section of the chapter.

Sample selection biases: orgasmic experience from coitus and masturbation

Tiefer (1992) has argued that Masters and Johnson's (1966) physiological research was not intended as an exploratory and open-minded inquiry into the possible range and diversity of human sexual response. (Indeed in chapter 5, I pointed out how Masters and Johnson (1966) did not properly investigate topics such as male multiple orgasm, male orgasm and ejaculation, and female ejaculation). According to Tiefer (1992), Masters and Johnson had very definite ideas about what kind of sexual responses they wanted to study even before they began their research. Their inquiry was limited from the outset by their requirement that all research subjects had to have a positive history of coital orgasm and masturbatory experience before they could be admitted into the research program (Masters and Johnson 1966, 311). Masters and Johnson were not interested in studying the sexual responses of subjects who did not regularly achieve orgasm via masturbation and coitus and so these people were arbitrarily excluded from the study. The researchers did admit some couples with sexual or conceptive problems but even these subjects presumably met the above entry requirement, otherwise they would not have been admitted (Masters and

Johnson 1966, 11, 312). This entry requirement seems to have been based on the assumption that sexual response normally leads to and includes orgasm. This means that Masters and Johnson's notion of a human sexual response cycle was assumed from the very outset of their research. It was not empirically discovered along the way as just one possible pattern of sexual response. Indeed, Masters and Johnson's research, which was based upon the responses of pre-selected orgasmic subjects, could do little else than to confirm the researchers' prior assumptions about human sexual response (Tiefer 1992, 234).

Masters once explained in an interview that the selection criterion of orgasmic experience was used because he and Johnson only wanted to study 'subjects who had a history of successful sexual response' ('Playboy Interview: Masters and Johnson' 1976, 140). He did not explain why he and Johnson thought that only sexual responses which lead to orgasm are successful and worthy of study. It is likely, however, that their goal-oriented view of sexual response was linked to their essentialist assumptions about human sexuality. In *Human Sexual Response*, for example, they wrote that orgasm was the ultimate end point of the human sexual response cycle and that it was generally thought to have developed from a deep biological-behavioural drive within the human species (Masters and Johnson 1966, 127).

For Masters and Johnson, 'successful' sexual response is sexual response which moves through a complete cycle from a state of quiescence through orgasm and back to quiescence. They even refer to their own research as being based on at least '10,000 *complete cycles* of sexual response for the total research population' (Masters and Johnson 1966, 15; emphasis added). Masters and Johnson attach the label 'successful' to those physiological changes in their research participants which accord with the researchers' own essentialist views about human sexual response. The research volunteers themselves were not asked what they considered to be 'successful' sexual response.

Masters and Johnson seem unaware that other people might not share their views about 'successful' sexual response or that they might even regard other kinds of sexual response as being 'successful.' Some evidence for this latter possibility is provided in a survey of sexual attitudes and lifestyles in Britain (Johnson et al 1994). This survey was based on a random sample of almost 19,000 people and included a section on attitudes about the relationship between orgasm and sexual satisfaction. 'Successful' sexual response, in this case, could conceivably be understood in terms of subjective judgements made about sexual satisfaction by the participants in the survey.

The study found that less than half (48.7%) of men surveyed agreed or strongly agreed that orgasm was essential for male sexual satisfaction. As many as a third (33.9%) of all men surveyed did not believe orgasm was necessary for male sexual satisfaction, and the remainder of men (17.4%)

neither agreed nor disagreed that orgasm was necessary. According to Anne Johnson et al (1994, 256), 'Orgasm is clearly not universally conceived as a prerequisite to male sexual satisfaction. This tends to run counter to the popular stereotype of men as sexually goal seeking.'

A similar situation held for women although there were gender differences in the proportions of men and women accepting or rejecting the necessity of orgasm for sexual satisfaction. Almost half (49.9%) of all women surveyed believed that sex without orgasm could be really satisfying for a woman while less than a third (28.6%) of women believed that orgasm was essential for female sexual satisfaction. The remaining women (21.5%) neither agreed nor disagreed about the necessity of orgasm for female satisfaction (Johnson et al 1994, 256).

In brief, sexual responses short of orgasm, which Masters and Johnson would regard as 'unsuccessful', could still be regarded as 'successful' (sexually satisfying) by a large proportion of the population (at least one-third of British men and almost one-half of British women in the sample). This means it would be unwise to use Masters and Johnson's (1966) model of the human sexual response cycle — based as it is on an essentialist goal-oriented view of sexuality, and an 'easily orgasmic sample' — to provide clinical norms of 'successful' (or 'healthy') sexual response for the general population (Tiefer 1992, 234). Masters and Johnson's view that 'successful' sexual response necessarily involves orgasm has more in common with popular ideology about male sexuality than with the more complex reality of men's and women's attitudes on the subject.

Tiefer (1992) has further argued that Masters and Johnson's (1966) decision to impose the same entry requirement of coital and masturbatory orgasmic experience on male and female research participants served to hide significant gender differences in experience with masturbation. Kinsey et al's (1953, 143) research, published just one year before Masters and Johnson's (1966) study began, found that '58 per cent of the females in our sample were masturbating to orgasm at some point in their lives.' By contrast, Kinsey et al (1948, 499) found that 'about 92 per cent of the total [male] population is involved in masturbation which leads to orgasm.' Kinsey et al's (1948; 1953) research was not based on a sample of people who were representative of U.S. society. However, in the absence of such research, it provides the best available survey evidence of sexual behaviour in the United States around the time when Masters and Johnson's research began. Kinsey et al's (1948;1953) research, even with its various limitations, suggests that Masters and Johnson's male research volunteers might have been more representative of males in the wider population than were their female volunteers of females in the general population. By imposing the same entry requirement on their male and female research participants, Masters and Johnson might have screened out important gender differences in masturbatory experience, and virtually ensured that their male and female volunteers produced the similar sexual responses which

Masters and Johnson later claimed was a major discovery of their work (Tiefer 1992, 234–5).

Sample selection biases: desire for effective sexual performance

Masters and Johnson (1966, 315) reported another significant difference between their research sample and the general population. Their research volunteers showed a pronounced desire to become effective sexual performers.

> Through the years of research exposure, the one factor in sexuality that consistently has been present among members of the study-subject population has been a basic interest in and desire for effectiveness of sexual performance. This one factor may represent the major area of difference between the research study subjects and the general population. (Masters and Johnson 1966, 315)

The research subjects' desire for and interest in effective sexual performance suggests that many of the subjects probably shared Masters and Johnson's view that sexual performance is effective when it leads to orgasm and the completion of the sexual response cycle. Masters and Johnson (1966, 315) suspect, however, that this view and motivation might not be so widely held in the general population. The previously cited study by Johnson et al (1994) suggests they could be right. Many people in the British survey believed that sexual satisfaction did not necessarily depend on what Masters and Johnson believed was 'effective sexual performance,' that is, orgasm and the completion of the sexual response cycle.

When substantial numbers of people place relatively less emphasis on goal-oriented sexual performance, then their motivation to pursue it is also likely to be less than that of Masters and Johnson's volunteers. Masters and Johnson's selection of sexual enthusiasts concerned with 'effective sexual performance' was probably at the expense of people who did not volunteer for their research but who had different views, motivations and sexual priorities when compared with Masters and Johnson's sample. The problem, once again, for Masters and Johnson's (1966) research is that this key difference is not adequately taken into account when their model of human sexual response is generalised as a set of clinical norms to the wider population. As Tiefer (1992, 236) points out, 'The consequences of choosing enthusiasts' values as the norm is to give the general population two choices — become enthusiasts, or suffer the opprobrium of official medical inadequacy.'

'The Bias of "Effective" Sexual Stimulation'

Masters and Johnson's (1966, 4) research was chiefly designed to discover the physical reactions of men and women in response to effective sexual stimulation. At no stage, however, do Masters and Johnson (1966) define what they mean by 'effective sexual stimulation.' According to Tiefer (1995, 48), 'The reader must discover that *"effective sexual stimulation"* is *that stimulation which facilitates a response that conforms to the HSRC* [human sexual response cycle]' (emphasis in original). She infers this from a close reading of the passages in *Human Sexual Response* where the term 'effective sexual stimulation' is used. She gives as an example a passage where Masters and Johnson reported on the sexual response of the labia minora to 'effective sexual stimulation.'

> Many women have progressed well into plateau-phase levels of sexual response, had the effective stimulative techniques withdrawn, and been unable to achieve orgasmic-phase tension release.... When an obviously effective means of sexual stimulation is withdrawn and orgasmic-phase release is not achieved, the minor-labial coloration will fade rapidly.... (Masters and Johnson 1966, 41–2)

This passage indicates that, for Masters and Johnson, the term 'effective sexual stimulation' means stimulation which produces physiological responses in conformity to the human sexual response cycle. Stimulation is labelled as 'effective' when it facilitates a progression through the stages of the sexual response cycle toward orgasm. If sexual stimulation does not lead to heightened sexual response then it is regarded as 'ineffective' and not worth studying (Tiefer 1995, 48). This adds weight to the argument that Masters and Johnson did not simply discover the human sexual response cycle during the course of their research. They assumed its 'truth' at the very outset of their investigation. They not only selected research subjects capable of, and enthusiastic about, performing to the requirements of this cycle but they narrowed their research interests to subjects' responses which conformed to it (Tiefer 1995, 48–9).

Experimenter bias in the research laboratory

'Experimenter biases' occur when researchers communicate their expectations to research participants and thereby influence the behaviour they wish to study. Experimenter biases seem to have occurred in Masters and Johnson's (1966) research both in the initial orientation program (Tiefer 1992, 236) and later during the actual research itself. These biases again highlight Masters and Johnson's pre-existing assumptions about human sexual response and the way these are implicated in the construction of their 'findings.'

Before Masters and Johnson's (1966, 22) empirical research on sexual physiology began, those volunteers selected as research subjects had to enter a preliminary orientation program. After providing their social, medical and sexual histories and undergoing physical examinations, the volunteers were introduced to the sex research laboratory and allowed time to adjust to their surroundings. Sexual activity was encouraged at first in private and later with the researchers present. The physical responses of subjects were not recorded until they felt at ease in the laboratory and were confident that they could sexually perform. Nevertheless, the highest number of sexual performance failures occurred during the orientation program (Masters and Johnson 1966, 313).

Masters and Johnson (1966, 313) were very clear on what constituted failures of sexual performance. Failures involved sexual responses without orgasm ('orgasmic inadequacy'); sexual responses where penile erection was not attained or maintained 'to a degree sufficient for mounting effectiveness' ('erective inadequacy'); and sexual responses involving fast male ejaculation which caused 'coital failure' ('premature ejaculation'). Masters and Johnson were not interested in studying 'failures' of sexual performance. Their research interest was in 'successful' sexual response which progressed from one stage of the sexual response cycle to the next, and which properly terminated in orgasm.

It seems that during the orientation program, Masters and Johnson communicated their views on what constituted 'successful' and 'unsuccessful' sexual performances to their research subjects. The subjects were likely to have been quite receptive to this information given that they were predominantly sexual enthusiasts who had volunteered their services. Research suggests that volunteer research subjects are also more receptive to cues from researchers than are non-volunteers (Tiefer 1992, 236).

Masters and Johnson (1966, 313) actually gave their subjects explicit advice on changing any 'problematic' sexual responses which occurred during the orientation period. They admit, for example, that:

> premature ejaculation occasionally has been a problem with *new* members of the male population. Fortunately, this sexual inadequacy has been readily reversible. *Premature ejaculation has not been of continuing concern, once adequate technical and clinical suggestions have been made, accepted and practiced.* (Masters and Johnson 1966, 313; emphasis added)

The same kind of experimenter biases seem to have occurred throughout the research, not just in the initial orientation period. Masters and Johnson (1966, 313) reported, for example, that there were 338 failures of coitus and masturbation in the research laboratory during the eleven year period in which they recorded at least ten thousand complete cycles of sexual response. When these 'failures' occurred, Masters and Johnson acted as educators and therapists to help their subjects produce more 'successful' sexual performances. 'When female orgasmic or male ejaculatory failures develop in the laboratory, the situation is discussed immediately. Once the individual has been reassured, suggestions are made for improvement of future performance' (Masters and Johnson 1966, 314).

In writing about their research program, Masters and Johnson (1966, 312) are quite open about the way in which their research actually affected the sexual responses they were studying. Indeed, they consider these effects to be positive because they conform to what they regard as 'effective' sexual response. 'After eleven years there was no information available to suggest that active cooperation with the investigation *has done other than maintain or improve the effectiveness of individual sexual expression*' (Masters and Johnson 1966, 312; emphasis added).

The upshot of this is that Masters and Johnson not only chose sexual enthusiasts keen to perform to their requirements; and not only narrowed their research interests to those 'successful' sexual responses which conformed to their pre-existing notion of a human sexual response cycle; but they even advised and coached subjects who could not 'successfully' perform in order to engineer the desired responses. This adds further weight to the argument that the human sexual response cycle is an inappropriate model for defining norms of sexual health and illness for the general population.

Sample selection biases: socioeconomic differences

Masters and Johnson's (1966) research sample was designed not to reflect a cross-section of the socioeconomic characteristics of U.S. society. They deliberately weighted their sample toward people of above average 'intelligence' and socioeconomic status; and they did not offset this group 'by a statistically significant number of lower-range family units'... (Masters and Johnson 1966, 11–12). In addition to this bias, Masters and Johnson (1966, 12) further narrowed their sample by using an interview to determine people's willingness to participate in the research, their capacity for sexual response, and their ability to communicate the specific details of their sexual reactions.

As discussed in chapter 4, Masters and Johnson did not believe that social differences between their study subjects and the general population had any bearing on their research into sexual physiology. Their belief was based on an essentialist assumption that the human body has a universal physical response to 'effective' sexual stimulation and that this would be unaffected by socioeconomic factors. Tiefer (1995, 45) points out, however, that 'The irony of assuming that physiology is universal and therefore that class (sic) differences make no difference is that no one conducts research that asks the question.'

Prior to Masters and Johnson's (1966) work, however, Kinsey et al's (1948;1953) research was partly concerned with how human sexual behaviour varies with socioeconomic status. They found wide differences in sexual behaviour between members of different socioeconomic groups, for example, in relation to masturbation, petting, oral-genital sex and the positions used in sexual intercourse. More importantly, however, they found that it was not just volitional sexual activity which was affected in this way by socioeconomic status.

Kinsey and his colleagues (1948, 343) commented, for example, that it was 'particularly interesting to find' that there were significant 'differences between educational levels in regard to nocturnal emissions — a type of sexual outlet which one might suppose would represent involuntary behaviour'. The researchers also found that nocturnal emissions varied with the occupational 'class' of the individual. There 'are 10 to 12 times as frequent nocturnal emissions among males of the upper occupational classes as there are among males of the lower classes' (Kinsey et al 1948, 345). The researchers were not sure how to explain these differences. They conjectured that they might be related to an individual's 'imaginative capacity' or the 'paucity of overt socio-sexual experience among upper level males [which] accounts both for their daytime eroticism and for their nocturnal dreaming' (Kinsey et al 1948, 345).

At the very least, this kind of evidence does suggest that social factors can influence human sexual response (even when it seems to be involuntary). The more that people from different socioeconomic backgrounds vary in their sexual responses from Masters and Johnson's (1966) narrow sample, the less Masters and Johnson's human sexual response cycle 'is appropriate as a universal norm' (Tiefer 1995, 45).

GENDER BIASES IN THE CLASSIFICATION OF SEXUAL DYSFUNCTION

Masters and Johnson's (1970) nosology of sexual dysfunction is largely based on their research into human sexual response. This research emphasised the similarities rather than the differences in male and female sexual response. Given this emphasis, it might be expected that the nosology, too, would emphasise the similarities in the types of sexual dysfunction experienced by men and women. In fact, however, as well as similarities, there are some important gender differences in the way that Masters and Johnson classified sexual dysfunctions.

Firstly, Masters and Johnson's (1970) nosology contains no female equivalent of the male sexual dysfunction premature ejaculation. The corresponding female dysfunction would presumably be 'premature orgasm.' This discrepancy means that premature ejaculation is only defined as a sexual dysfunction in men whereas premature orgasm in women is not defined as a disorder at all. Masters and Johnson, in effect, have judged the similar sexual functioning of men and women ('fast' ejaculation/orgasm) by entirely different standards. They did not attempt to explain or justify this double standard. They simply imposed it.

Many years later, however, Masters et al (1985) introduced the undefined category of 'rapid orgasm' as the female counterpart of premature ejaculation. They said that rapid orgasm 'has been almost completely ignored by sexologists. This is probably because this condition is relatively rare. In more than two decades of our research, we have encountered only a handful of women who complained of reaching orgasm too quickly' (Masters et al 1985, 503–4).

Masters et al's (1985) comments above suggest that the reason they *might* not have originally included the category of female rapid orgasm in their (1970) nosology was because fast female orgasm is a rare phenomenon. If this is the explanation, there are two problems with it. Firstly, there is evidence that it may not be as rare as Masters et al (1985) believe. Frank et al (1978), for example, surveyed 100 married couples about their experience of sexual dysfunction. These couples were not seeking help for sexual or marital problems at the time of the survey. Frank et al (1978) found that 11% of the females complained of reaching orgasm 'too quickly.' More recently, Laumann et al (1994, 371) reported the results from a survey of sexual practices. The survey used a probability sample of 1,623 American women between the ages of 18 and 59. Laumann et al (1994) found that 10.3% of women surveyed reported climaxing 'too quickly.'

Secondly, there is the question of whether the rarity of a pathological condition is sufficient justification for not classifying it. Leaving aside the question of whether rapid orgasm is a pathological condition, it is unlikely that medical scientists would not classify a pathological condition just because it occurred infrequently. It is similarly difficult to believe that Masters and Johnson, who worked within the medical model, did not classify rapid orgasm as a dysfunction simply because they believed it rarely occurred. After all, Masters and Johnson, by their own admission, classified a number of other infrequently occurring sexual dysfunctions. For example, they included 'ejaculatory incompetence' in their nosology even though they saw only seventeen men complaining of this in eleven years (Masters and Johnson 1970, 116). They also included female 'masturbatory orgasmic inadequacy' in the nosology while admitting they only saw eleven women seeking help for this in the same period (Masters and Johnson 1970, 248). Similarly, they suggested that 'low sexual tension' be considered as a potential clinical entity even though they acknowledged that it rarely occurred or was professionally identified (Masters and Johnson 1970, 247). In actual fact, they had only one case history that they thought might fit this diagnostic category.

Masters and Johnson (1970) seem to have regarded premature ejaculation as a sexual dysfunction because they assumed that women must reach a climax by prolonged penile thrusting in their vaginas. They believed that premature ejaculation is a dysfunction because it prevents female orgasm from occurring. Accordingly, in their view, men must learn to control their ejaculations until their female partners climax. They do not acknowledge that after ejaculation men might be willing and able to sexually satisfy their partners. By contrast, Masters and Johnson did not regard rapid female orgasm as a dysfunction because they thought it did not prevent a woman's male partner from reaching orgasm through penile movement in her vagina. They assumed that after a woman has a 'rapid orgasm' she will continue sexual intercourse until her male partner is sexually satisfied. Accordingly, in Masters and Johnson's view, there would be no reason for a female to control her orgasm until her male partner climaxed (Masters et al 1985, 504).

Masters et al (1985, 504) later noted, however, that at least some women who have a 'rapid orgasm' do lose interest in further sexual activity and may find it physically uncomfortable. This seems to be the reason they belatedly included the category of 'rapid orgasm' in their nosology. This inclusion, however, was only temporary because the category had again disappeared by the time of their later work *Heterosexuality* (1994).

Apart from the gender bias in Masters and Johnson's (1970) nosology concerning fast ejaculation or orgasm, there is also the important question of whether premature ejaculation or rapid orgasm are pathological conditions at all. I have argued elsewhere that 'premature ejaculation' seems to be a 'socially constructed' problem rather than a form of pathology (Morrow 1994; Morrow 2005). It rarely, if ever, has an organic cause and it is not usually associated with illness, disease or disability. It even conforms to Masters and Johnson's own model of the human sexual response cycle with effective sexual stimulation producing ejaculation. However, it is a type of sexual response which deviates from social expectations about how much time it should take men to ejaculate during coitus. If social norms encourage 'fast' male ejaculation (as, for example, in East Bay, Melanesia), then ejaculations which take too long can be seen as problematic, and may be pathologised as 'retarded ejaculations' (Davenport 1968, 217; Reiss 1986, 238). However, when social norms encourage 'slow' male ejaculation, (for example, in many contemporary Western societies), then ejaculations which happen too quickly are pathologised as 'early' or 'premature' ejaculations. In other words, the very same sexual response, and the same amount of time taken to ejaculate, can be regarded as healthy or normal by one set of social norms, and unhealthy or abnormal by another. Masters et al (1985) did not define the category of rapid orgasm in women. However, if it is defined in a similar way to premature ejaculation, then similar criticisms would probably apply to it.

The second gender bias in Masters and Johnson's (1970) nosology of sexual dysfunction is that there is no female dysfunction equivalent to male impotence. That is, Masters and Johnson do not have a category of sexual dysfunction which refers to disorders of sexual arousal in women (Wakefield 1987, 468). Masters and Johnson (1970, 247–8) did suggest a female category of 'low sexual tension' as a 'potential clinical entity' but 'it is clear from the one case described that this does not necessarily refer to pre-orgasmic responses, in the way that impotence clearly does' (Boyle 1994, 109–10). Boyle (1994, 109) argues that the omission of a female category analogous to impotence is difficult to justify because Masters and Johnson's (1966) own research emphasised the essential similarity of male and female sexual response. Both sexes experience vasocongestion during sexual arousal but Masters and Johnson (1970) only regarded the lack of vasocongestion in men as a sexual dysfunction. They did not explain why they omitted an equivalent category for women.

The clear gender bias in their classification of sexual arousal disorders has a number of important consequences. Firstly, it creates a gender bias in the diagnosis of sexual arousal disorders. Masters and Johnson (1970) logically discriminated between disorders of arousal and disorders of orgasm in men but not in women. This means that a man who fails to experience sexual arousal can be diagnosed as impotent under Masters and Johnson's (1970) nosology but a woman in the same situation cannot be given an equivalent diagnosis. In their sex therapy program, Masters and Johnson (1970) actually diagnosed such women as suffering from disorders of orgasm (primary orgasmic dysfunction) (Wakefield 1987, 468). As Wakefield (1987, 468) points out, however, 'It makes no more sense to diagnose an arousal problem in a woman as an orgasmic disorder than it would to diagnose an impotent man as ejaculatorily incompetent.' It also unjustifiably tends to inflate the number of women believed to suffer from primary orgasmic dysfunction (Wakefield 1987, 468).

Secondly, the gender bias in the classification of sexual arousal disorders makes it seem that male genital swelling is more important than its female counterpart. According to Boyle (1993, 81), however:

> It is more important that men experience genital swelling during sexual encounters only if we believe that the act of penetration is the most important outcome. Women can, after all, participate in, or be subjected to, intercourse without experiencing genital swelling, particularly if an artificial lubricant is used. To pay more attention to male vasocongestion not only makes intercourse central, but reflects the cultural stereotype of women as the recipients of male action and desire, but whose own desire is secondary.

Thirdly, the omission of a category for the lack of female vasocongestion may serve to deny or invalidate women's own experiences of this phenomenon. It also restricts the development of a language with which women can think about their sexual responses and communicate with others (Boyle 1993, 81).

Finally, the lack of attention to female vasocongestion has impeded research into the phenomenon. Research 'on the effects of drugs and disease on male vasocongestion far exceeds research on their effects on women' (Boyle 1993, 82).

In the light of these criticisms, one might have expected that Masters and Johnson would have amended their nosology to remove the gender bias in the classification of sexual arousal disorders. However, in the case of these disorders, Masters et al (1985; 1994) continued to reproduce the same biased nosology that they introduced in 1970.

The third gender bias in Masters and Johnson's (1970) nosology is that there is no male dysfunction which corresponds to female primary orgasmic dysfunction. That is, they do not have a diagnostic category that specifically refers to the total and lifelong inability of men to experience orgasm. Masters and Johnson do have a category of 'ejaculatory incompetence' but this only refers to a man's inability to ejaculate during coitus. This dysfunction is really the equivalent of female 'coital orgasmic dysfunction.' Since Masters and Johnson conflated orgasm and ejaculation in men, and did not recognise female ejaculation, the lack of male ejaculation can be regarded in their nosology as equivalent to the lack of female orgasm.

The result of this asymmetrical classification is that men and women with the same experience — a lack of orgasm from masturbation and coitus — would be diagnosed differently depending on their gender. Women would be diagnosed with primary orgasmic dysfunction while there is no equivalent diagnosis for men. In Masters and Johnson's male clinical population, such men were diagnosed with ejaculatory incompetence even though they did not fit this category because they could not ejaculate from coitus or masturbation (Masters et al 1985, 499).

Wakefield (1987, 467) suggests that the male equivalent of primary orgasmic dysfunction might conveniently be called 'total ejaculatory incompetence.' By extrapolating from Masters and Johnson's definitions of ejaculatory incompetence he offers a definition of total ejaculatory incompetence. 'Total ejaculatory incompetence is the inability to ejaculate during sexual activity, including both intercourse and masturbation, despite having a sufficiently firm erection and relatively high levels of sexual arousal' (Wakefield 1987, 467). By contrast, Masters et al (1985, 502) said that '*Primary anorgasmia* refers to women who have never had an orgasm' (emphasis in original). 'In order to be diagnosed as having primary orgasmic dysfunction, a woman must report lack of orgasmic attainment during her entire lifespan' (Masters and Johnson 1970, 227).

When the rates of men and women experiencing total ejaculatory incompetence and primary orgasmic dysfunction, respectively, are compared in Masters and Johnson's (1970) clinical population an interesting finding emerges. Only 0.5% of the 448 men seeking therapy could not ejaculate from either masturbation or coitus (but had experienced nocturnal emissions) (Masters et al 1985, 499). By contrast, Masters and Johnson (1970, 239) diagnosed 56% of the 342 women in their clinical population as having primary orgasmic dysfunction (including two women who had experienced orgasms in dreams or fantasy but not from physical stimulation) (Masters and Johnson 1970, 227). '*This means that the rate of POD* [primary orgasmic dysfunction] *in women was over 100 times the rate of its male equivalent in Masters and Johnson's clinical population'* (Wakefield 1987, 466; emphasis in original).

Wakefield (1987) argues that the enormous disparity in the diagnostic rates of primary orgasmic dysfunction and total ejaculatory incompetence can be partly explained by the gender bias in the diagnostic criteria of the relevant categories. Primary orgasmic dysfunction is an inherently broader category than total ejaculatory incompetence in two main ways. Firstly, women who have never had an orgasm can be diagnosed with primary orgasmic dysfunction even if they have never engaged in sexual activities, such as masturbation and coitus. Similarly, women who have not orgasmed because they have never received adequate sexual stimulation would also fit the category of primary orgasmic dysfunction. In other words, women who may have an ability to orgasm but who have not achieved it through lack of learning, opportunity or stimulation would still be regarded as having primary orgasmic dysfunction. However, the same is not true for men. Men would only be diagnosed with total ejaculatory incompetence if they could not ejaculate *during* sexual activities, such as intercourse and masturbation, in which they received 'adequate' sexual stimulation. A man who had not had an orgasm because he had never tried intercourse or masturbation or because he did not receive sufficient sexual stimulation would not be diagnosed with total ejaculatory incompetence (Wakefield 1987, 467–8).

Secondly, women who do not orgasm because they have not become highly aroused would be diagnosed with primary orgasmic dysfunction but men in the same situation would *not* be diagnosed with total ejaculatory incompetence. If a man is not sexually aroused enough to have a firm erection, then Masters and Johnson would diagnose his dysfunction as impotence. By contrast, they diagnosed women who lacked high arousal as having orgasm disorders because there was no available category of female dysfunction equivalent to impotence. In sum, many more women were diagnosed with primary orgasmic dysfunction than would have occurred if the category of primary orgasmic dysfunction had the same diagnostic criteria as total ejaculatory incompetence (Wakefield 1987, 468–9). According to Wakefield (1987, 469):

> the nonspecific criteria for female orgasmic dysfunctions implies that many other problems, such as disorders of desire and even vaginismus, will end up being engulfed by the category of orgasmic dysfunction and increase the female rate of diagnosis. This biased construction of diagnostic criteria explains the otherwise amazing fact that *every single woman* in Masters and Johnson's clinical sample was diagnosed as having some kind of orgasmic disorder. (emphasis in original)

The final gender bias in Masters and Johnson's (1970) nosology is that there is no male dysfunction equivalent to female 'situational orgasmic dysfunction.' Only women are regarded as dysfunctional if they have had at least one orgasm but otherwise have difficulties reaching orgasm. Men in the same situation would not be regarded as having a sexual dysfunction. Masters and Johnson divided situational orgasmic dysfunction into three subcategories: masturbatory orgasmic inadequacy, coital orgasmic inadequacy and random orgasmic inadequacy. Coital orgasmic inadequacy corresponds to the male dysfunction ejaculatory incompetence. However, there is no male dysfunction equivalent to masturbatory orgasmic inadequacy. Only women are considered to be dysfunctional if they cannot orgasm from masturbation but can orgasm from coitus. Men in the same situation would not be regarded as having a dysfunction. Similarly, there is no male dysfunction which corresponds to random orgasmic inadequacy. Only women can be diagnosed with this dysfunction. Men who have had an orgasm at least once from masturbation and coitus but who otherwise are rarely orgasmic and have little need for sexual expression would not be considered dysfunctional.

THE HETERO-COITAL BIAS OF THE NOSOLOGY

I have argued elsewhere that although Masters and Johnson (1970) transplanted their model of the human sexual response cycle from the laboratory to the clinical context, their nosology of sexual dysfunction is not solely based on the explicit version of this model (Morrow 1996, 170). In its explicit form the human sexual response cycle is an asocial model of sexual response which only refers to the similar sexual responses of individual male and female bodies. In the clinical context, however, Masters and Johnson (1970, 3) wanted to treat *marital relationships* as their patients, not simply individuals. In focusing on marital relationships it was not sufficient to simply diagnose and treat isolated individuals whose sexual responses deviated from the human sexual response cycle. Masters and Johnson had to consider sexual response within a social context where spouses were sexually interacting. This is where the implicit essentialist and hetero-coital assumptions of the human sexual response cycle model become more evident.

Masters and Johnson assumed that normal sexual response developed from an underlying sex drive and was the body's involuntary preparation for heterosexual coitus (penis in vagina sex). They implicitly believed that heterosexual coitus was the 'natural' form of sexual interaction between male and female partners (as did probably most of their clients) and that marital relationships were threatened if spouses could not have 'sex' in this 'normal' way. Consequently, their (1970) nosology of sexual dysfunction is overwhelmingly concerned with problems of genital functioning which impede the 'effective' physical performance of heterosexual coitus (Morrow 1996, 170).

The first problem with making the 'satisfactory' performance of heterosexual coitus the universal standard of healthy sexual functioning is that all those who cannot perform this activity would appear to be sexually dysfunctional by definition. The psychoanalyst, Irving Bieber, has said, for example, that homosexuals should be regarded as sexually dysfunctional on the grounds that they cannot function heterosexually (Soble 1987, 117–19). It was previously argued, however, that Masters and Johnson's essentialist view of sexuality, and the research based on this, was unable to adequately explain how heterosexual coitus constituted the natural and universal purpose of human sexual response. This means that the choice of heterosexual coitus as the standard of healthy sexual functioning is actually relative to the dominant values of social groups. Coitus not only 'constitutes the truth of sexuality in the public common-sense of the west' (Matthews 1992, 125) but it 'has always held a privileged position in western ideology' (Berg 1986, 168). If coitus is not taken 'as a universal standard of "normal" sexual functioning but as an activity that is valued by a particular', if very large, part of the population, 'then those who are not heterosexual need not be judged in terms of this particular activity' (Morrow 2005, 193).

The second problem with using heterosexual coitus as the standard of healthy sexual functioning is that it ignores known and relevant differences between men's and women's sexual functioning in this type of activity. More specifically, men and women have differential access to achieving orgasm from penile movement in the vagina (Myerson 1986, 68; Morrow 1994, 26). Heterosexual men are generally able to reach orgasm in the vast majority of their coital activity but the same is not generally true for women (Kinsey et al 1953, 371, 393). Research by Hite (1989) and Berg (1986), for example, indicates that most women do not orgasm from penile movement in the vagina alone. The main reason for this is that (other things being equal) the man is usually receiving direct stimulation of his penis, and may also be controlling the depth, angle, rhythm and speed of the thrusting to suit his own needs, while the woman may, at best, only be experiencing indirect stimulation of her clitoris (the main site of her erotic sensitivity) (Hite 1989, 276). In this scenario, it is not surprising that men will reach orgasm faster and more consistently than women. This corresponds with Kaplan's (1978, 282) view that, when considering the frequency of sexual dysfunctions, failure to orgasm 'is relatively rare in men, in contrast, it is the most common sexual complaint of women.' Masters et al (1985, 505) themselves estimate that less than five per cent of all cases of female anorgasmia (failure to orgasm) have organic causes.

In non-coital sexual activities, however, women do not necessarily 'take longer to orgasm than men' (Hite 1989, 269), and the vast majority of women in both the Kinsey and Hite reports masturbated not by using vaginal entry techniques but by clitoral and/or labial stimulation (Gould 1991, 129). It is only when women experience indirect and insufficient stimulation in activities like coitus that they have more difficulty in reaching orgasm.

The problem, then, of using a hetero-coital standard of sexual health is that it fails to take into account known gender differences in sexual functioning during this activity. This can lead to the pathologisation of otherwise normal women as orgasmically dysfunctional (Morrow 1994, 26–8).

The third problem with the hetero-coital bias of Masters and Johnson's (1970) nosology is that, in general, genital performance is only regarded as a dysfunction if it impedes the enactment of penis in vagina sex (Morrow 1996, 171). If the same genital performances occur during non hetero-coital sex then they usually do not count as dysfunctions in Masters and Johnson's (1970) nosology. For example, 'fast' ejaculation, lack of ejaculation, lack of erection and male genital pain are generally regarded as sexual dysfunctions only within the context of heterosexual intercourse. If they occur, for example, during masturbation, oral or anal intercourse then they are not usually considered dysfunctions. Similarly for women, vaginal spasms and genital pain are only defined as dysfunctions if they occur during heterosexual intercourse. If they occur during other sexual activities they are not regarded as dysfunctions. Lack of female orgasm is also primarily, but not exclusively, defined as a dysfunction during penis in vagina sex (Masters and Johnson 1970).

The main exception to the hetero-coital bias of the nosology is the female dysfunction 'masturbatory orgasmic inadequacy' (Morrow 1996, 171). This is not defined in relation to heterosexual coitus but its socially constructed nature is still clear. During the age of masturbatory insanity (Hare 1962), masturbation was considered to be a disease and not masturbating was the treatment. In this social context, Masters and Johnson's category of 'masturbatory orgasmic inadequacy' would have made little sense. Lack of masturbation to orgasm only became a problem when people changed their views about masturbation and began to regard it as a healthy and desirable activity (Szasz 1981, 64–5).

In more recent publications, Masters et al (1985; 1994) dropped the category of female masturbatory orgasmic inadequacy from their nosology of sexual dysfunction. They also made other changes, such as including a new category of male dysfunction called 'retarded ejaculation.' The new nosologies, however, continue to define genital performance dysfunctions only or primarily in relation to heterosexual coitus.

THE OMISSION OF PROBLEMS WITH SEXUAL DESIRE

Masters and Johnson's (1970) nosology of sexual dysfunction is exclusively concerned with 'problems' of physical performance. It does not encompass problems related to sexual desire. This is probably not surprising given that Masters and Johnson (1966) ignored the issue of sexual desire in favour of a sex drive underpinning for human sexual response (Morrow 1996). However, in the mid-1970s Harold Lief (1977) realised that many patients requesting treatment from sex therapy clinics could not be adequately diagnosed using Masters and Johnson's (1970) categories of sexual dysfunction. He suggested that the category of 'inhibited sexual desire' be included in the nosology of sexual dysfunctions. This category was meant to apply to patients who had a chronic inability to commence or respond to sexual stimulation. Helen Kaplan (1977) also believed that many of the treatment failures of sex therapy resulted from the lack of therapeutic attention to problems of 'hypoactive sexual desire.' She criticised Masters and Johnson's model of the human sexual response cycle and argued for a triphasic model of sexual response with sexual desire as the first and most important part of sexual arousal.

In their later work, Masters and Johnson acknowledged that their model of the human sexual response cycle was deficient in not including a phase of sexual desire (Masters et al 1994, 46). Since the mid-1970s they also accepted that people can have problems with sexual desire although they classified these problems separately from sexual dysfunctions (Masters et al (1985, 509).

THE MEDICALISATION OF DEVIANT SEXUAL RESPONSE

Masters and Johnson's (1970) nosology of sexual dysfunction is based on the assumption that those conditions which vary from their model of the human sexual response cycle are diseases (Lehrman 1976, 101–2). They define these conditions as diseases on the grounds that the human sexual response cycle represents healthy sexual functioning, that some of these variant conditions *are* caused by specific organic or psychosocial factors or because there is a suspicion that such factors might one day be found. They seem to assume that if conditions which are sometimes caused by such factors can occur independently of them then these conditions must be intrinsically pathological or else a manifestation of an as yet undiscovered form of pathology (Masters et al 1985, 504–5).

This medicalisation of deviant sexual response prepared the way for and legitimised the development of sex therapy as a new 'profession.' Since *Human Sexual Inadequacy* was published in 1970, an entire industry of sex clinics, therapists and counsellors has emerged to treat sexual dysfunctions in the population. Without denying that sexual responses might deviate from the human sexual response cycle, it is not clear that these deviations should be automatically regarded as pathological (Morrow 1996, 172–3). As Rowland (1999, 13) points out, Masters and Johnson's (1966) laboratory research was primarily concerned with establishing typical physiological responses to sexual stimulation. It was much less concerned with describing variations in sexual response or in accounting for those variations. Furthermore, in understanding variations in sexual response, it is very important to consider the social context within which it occurs.

This means that 'deviant' sexual responses, which Masters and Johnson think of as diseases, might be caused by disease or they might not. If a man is unable to maintain an erection during sex with his wife because he is bored after a long marriage, this does not seem to be a health problem. There 'is nothing biologically wrong with a male that will not respond to another repetition of the same stimulus' (Soble 1987, 119). Similarly, if a woman is unable to orgasm during sex with her husband because he does not provide her with adequate stimulation then this also does not seem to be a health problem (Soble 1987, 119). Masters et al (1985, 504) themselves state that eighty to ninety per cent of dysfunctions have no organic cause and their own version of sex therapy mainly involves 'treating' individuals who do not have an identifiable organic basis for their sexual dysfunctions. Nor is it clear that variations in sexual response are necessarily the result of defective psychological mechanisms or processes. Yet, if sex therapists and doctors define people's variations in sexual response as health or medical problems, and have these definitions accepted on the basis of their scientific or medical authority, then this territory has effectively been captured for the professional and material interests of these groups (Soble 1987, 119). Medicalisation is also bound up with social control as therapists seek to promote conformity to socially constructed norms of sexual functioning, and by pathologising and 'treating' responses which deviate from these norms (Morrow 1994).

THE CONFLATION OF SEXUAL DYSFUNCTIONS WITH SEXUAL PROBLEMS

Masters and Johnson's (1970) nosology of sexual dysfunction relies on the assumption that the conditions labelled as sexual dysfunctions are intrinsically problems for those who are experiencing them. This is because the conditions are deviations from an 'objectively' established model of normal sexual response, and are impediments to healthy sexual functioning, understood as the ability to perform heterosexual coitus. Masters and Johnson generally assume that experts, such as themselves, can define and classify such dysfunctions without reference to the subjective meaning these conditions might have for those who manifest them. The researchers tend to assume that individuals are sexually satisfied when their bodies, particularly their genitals, are in 'good' mechanical working order and that conversely, individuals are unhappy when their genitals 'malfunction.' This assumption is no doubt reasonable in many cases, but the problem with it is that subjective sexual satisfaction can vary independently of the conditions conceptualised as sexual dysfunctions. That is, individuals might be sexually satisfied even though their genitals could be regarded as dysfunctional in terms of Masters and Johnson's (1970) nosology; conversely, individuals might have fully functioning genitals and yet be sexually unhappy or distressed (Morrow 1996, 173–4).

The language of sex therapy tends to hide this insight. Within the field of sex therapy the narrower term 'sexual dysfunction' is often used as a synonym or substitute for the wider term 'sexual problem' (Mahoney 1983, 557). The danger in using the narrower term is that it gives the impression that sexual problems are identical with physical performance problems. Without denying that people can find their physical performances problematic, not everyone regards sexual dysfunctions as problems. Nor do all of those who define themselves as having sexual problems necessarily have physical performance problems. Consider the case of impotence. While impotence might seem to be a self-evident sexual problem, a man does not necessarily need an erect penis to experience sexual pleasure, orgasm or ejaculation. Nor does he necessarily need an erection to sexually please his partner (Morrow 1994, 30–1). As one man reported to Hite (1981, 351), for example, lack of erection is a:

> problem, only if we so define it. If (as is true) I don't need erection for arousal and orgasm; and if (as is true) the woman doesn't need my erection for her arousal and orgasm; then why is it a problem?...It is only a problem if we are blindly insistent on penis-vagina intercourse as essential.

The same is true for female dysfunctions like vaginismus. This might also seem to be an intrinsic sexual problem but a woman does not necessarily need a penetrable vagina to experience sexual pleasure or orgasm, and an impenetrable vagina does not necessarily prevent her from giving sexual pleasure to her partner (Ussher and Baker 1993, 4; Keystone 1994). The same points could be made about the other conditions listed as dysfunctions in Masters and Johnson's (1970) nosology.

At the heart of many of these judgements about defective sexual physiology is a hetero-coital model of sexuality. If this model of correct sexual functioning ceased to be dominant, and the coital imperative became optional, then many of these apparent sexual dysfunctions would disappear along with the culturally induced fears and anxieties that accompany them (Jeffreys 1990, 32). A woman would be much less likely to be sexually unresponsive or anorgasmic if there was no insistence that penis-in-vagina sex should be her sole or primary means of reaching orgasm or of judging her sexual functioning. A man would similarly feel much less pressure to produce an elusive vaginal orgasm with its accompanying requirements of a mandatory durable erection and ongoing efforts to delay his own climax. Similarly, a man (and his partner) would be much less likely to feel concerned about the timing of his ejaculation if there were acceptable options other than vaginal intercourse to provide his partner with sexual stimulation and orgasm. The same would be true in relation to vaginismus as pointed out above. In Western ideology, however, the dominance of the coital imperative has been achieved at the expense and subordination of other varieties of sexual interaction. These have historically been censured and condemned as sinful, immoral, sick and illegal (Morrow 1994, 31). While there seems to have been more exploration of non-coital sexuality since the time of Kinsey, coitus still remains the central sexual practice and 'most often both partners want orgasm in coitus' (Reiss 1986, 238; Berg 1986, 169–70; Bancroft 1989, 255; Laumann et al 1994; de Visser 2003).

One reason that people might think sexual dysfunctions are problems in themselves is because they have accepted the dominant cultural view that sex is the physical performance of coitus to orgasm, and that other sexual activities, if not actually 'deviant', are just preludes to, or embellishments of, the central sexual act. Yet as Mahoney (1983, 554) points out, even in the absence of genital functioning:

> people can still think about, touch, love, communicate with and appreciate another person. These core characteristics of sexuality do not require an erection, a moist vagina, erect clitoris, orgasm or the ability to position two bodies in a particular fashion so that they may move in unison in a certain manner.

Masters and Johnson's (1966) own narrow conceptualisation of human sexual response in terms of physiology was connected to their view that sexual problems are essentially sexual dysfunctions. When they began their laboratory research into human sexual physiology, they already believed, without providing empirical evidence, that sexual dysfunctions were the main cause of sexual dissatisfaction and the break-up of heterosexual marriages (Masters and Johnson 1966, vi). Subsequent research by Frank et al (1978), Waterman and Chiauzzi (1982) and Heiman et al (1986) has failed to find a significant correlation between sexual dysfunction and marital discontent. Masters and Johnson (1966) nevertheless argued that research into normal human sexual response was important in order to develop a baseline against which abnormal responses could be compared.

Masters and Johnson (1966) did not begin their research by asking men and women what they thought and felt about 'sex,' what they liked and did not like, and what they found to be problematic. Masters and Johnson were barely interested in the subjective dimension of sex. Their main priority was the observation and measurement of 'objective' physiological data. They could then use this data to define what was normal and what was abnormal so that the abnormal could be brought within the 'therapeutic gaze.' Lay people could then be expected to locate and understand their own sexual experiences within a 'scientifically' derived framework for determining health and illness. Had Masters and Johnson begun their research by asking people what they thought were sexual problems, the researchers might have come to a broader understanding of such problems and have been less inclined to reduce them to problems of physical performance (Morrow 1996, 175).

There seem to be few studies which actually ask people to define sexual problems in their own terms (Tiefer 1988, 12). Shere Hite is one of the few researchers to have done this. In her (1989) report on female sexuality, for example, women identified a variety of sexual problems not involving sexual dysfunction:

'I would like more love and gentleness instead of bare sexual stimulation — more emotion and communication...' (p. 530).

'More kisses, more time, more tenderness' (p. 530).

'More passion' (p. 531).

'I would like to have leisurely sex with a man more often, talking and fooling around and entertaining each other' (p. 531).

Some of the men in Hite's (1981) study of male sexuality also identified sexual problems which did not necessarily involve sexual dysfunction:

'Sex above all needs to be more...relaxed' (p. 339).

'Sexual intercourse with my wife has become unfortunately routine' (p. 415).

'My wife tends to want to rush things for my taste sometimes' (p. 421).

'I get virtually no foreplay from my partner, even when I ask for it' (p. 553).

These brief quotations from the female and male respondents to Hite's (1989; 1981) questionnaires indicate a range of sexual dissatisfactions which cannot be understood simply in terms of Masters and Johnson's concept or nosology of sexual dysfunction (Morrow 1996, 176). If, despite these self-identified sexual problems, Hite's respondents were physically functioning in accordance with the human sexual response cycle, and the requirements of heterosexual coitus, then their problems could not be recognised or given any legitimacy in terms of Masters and Johnson's previous or current nosologies of sexual dysfunction (Masters and Johnson 1970; Masters et al 1985; Tiefer 1988; Masters et al 1994).

CONCLUSION

Masters and Johnson's concept and classification of sexual dysfunction have been very influential within the fields of sexology and sex therapy. However, they have attracted relatively little criticism, probably because they are believed to be based on objective scientific data, and are compatible with dominant Western beliefs and values about sexuality.

This chapter provided a critique of their concept and classification of sexual dysfunction. The chapter began by discussing how Masters and Johnson's standard of healthy sexual functioning was partly based on the smooth mechanical functioning of the body, in accordance with their model of the human sexual response cycle. When they defined their concept of sexual dysfunction in relation to this norm, it referred to mechanical breakdowns in genital functioning and ineffective sexual performance. After outlining Masters and Johnson's (1970) new nosology of sexual dysfunction — probably the first since the Middle Ages — the chapter then discussed its perceived advantages over the earlier classification of sexual dysfunctions into impotence and frigidity.

The chapter then provided a critique of the major flaws in Masters and Johnson's nosology of sexual dysfunction. Firstly, drawing primarily on Tiefer's (1992) work, the chapter argued that Masters and Johnson's nosology was partly developed in relation to a model of healthy sexual functioning (the human sexual response cycle) which has limited generalisability in providing a set of clinical norms for the whole population.

Secondly, the chapter pointed out that since Masters and Johnson's (1966) research on sexual physiology had emphasised the sexual similarities between males and females, it might have been expected that their nosology of sexual dysfunction would contain similar types of sexual dysfunctions for males and females. While there were some similarities, the chapter also identified a number of gender biases in the classification of sexual dysfunction. In many cases, Masters and Johnson did not explain these gender asymmetries or why a particular kind of response is a dysfunction in one sex but not in the other. It was argued that these asymmetries can also have important consequences, for example, in the way that sexual dysfunctions are diagnosed and treated.

Thirdly, the chapter examined how Masters and Johnson's nosology of sexual dysfunction was developed in relation to a norm of healthy sexual functioning. This was partly based on the ability to 'satisfactorily' engage in hetero-coital sex. The adoption of this particular conception of sexuality as the norm of healthy sexual functioning appears to pathologise homosexual sexual response, and female inability to reach orgasm during coitus. It also marginalises non hetero-coital forms of sexual activity and largely excludes the possibility that sexual dysfunctions might occur during such activity.

Fourthly, the chapter argued that Masters and Johnson's nosology of sexual dysfunction is exclusively concerned with problems of physical performance during sexual activity and has no scope for dealing with possible problems concerning sexual desire. This was probably not surprising given that they ignored the issue of sexual desire in their model of the human sexual response cycle.

Fifthly, the chapter explained how Masters and Johnson tended to regard physiological deviations from their model of sexual response as diseases. This medicalisation of deviant sexual response legitimised and prepared the way for sex therapy as a new 'profession' and institution of social control. The chapter argued, however, that physiological deviations from the model of the human sexual response cycle are not necessarily signs of pathology.

Finally, I argued that Masters and Johnson tended to conflate the terms 'sexual dysfunction' and 'sexual problem.' This led, on the one hand, to a neglect of the way that people did not always regard sexual dysfunctions as sexual problems. On the other hand, it led to a narrow focus on inabilities of physical performance, and a neglect of any broader understanding of what people might regard as sexual problems.

However, despite the various defects in Masters and Johnson's nosology, it played a central role in the development of their 'new' sex therapy program. The following chapter examines the nature of this program, and provides a critique of its principles, practices and reported effectiveness.

7 A Critique of Masters and Johnson's Sex Therapy Program

INTRODUCTION

Masters and Johnson's (1970) second book, *Human Sexual Inadequacy*, not only provided a new nosology of sexual dysfunction, it also described the principles and practices of their sex therapy program, and results from eleven years of clinical treatment and five years of patient follow-up. The book claimed to provide a new way of treating sexual dysfunctions which was brief and intensive with a low rate of treatment failure. This book helped to launch the new 'profession' of sex therapy. Its claims were widely accepted for many years and most sex therapists still draw, to a greater or lesser extent, on Masters and Johnson's 'pioneering' work.

This chapter aims to critically review the nature and results of Masters and Johnson's therapy program. It will be argued that the therapy program is underpinned by problematic concepts of sexual function and dysfunction; that the discussion of the aetiology of sexual dysfunction ignores the social and political context of sexual functioning; that their therapeutic methods have limited usefulness in resolving many of the problems experienced by heterosexual patients; that their goal of returning sex to its natural context is misconceived and unattainable; that their claims of treatment efficacy could not be replicated because they provided insufficient information about their treatment program; that their therapy program operates as an institution of social control which promotes conformity to a hetero-coital model of sexual functioning; and that many of their therapeutic claims were uncritically accepted on the basis of their past research, scientific reputations, and the indebtedness of sexologists to their 'pioneering' work.

The chapter begins, however, with a discussion of the origin of their therapy program and their concept of sex as a natural function.

MASTERS AND JOHNSON'S SEX THERAPY PROGRAM

On the basis of their laboratory research, Masters and Johnson developed a clinical program for the treatment of sexual dysfunction. This program began in 1959 in a clinic at Washington University. It was 'transferred to the Reproductive Biology Research Foundation in 1964' (Masters and Johnson 1970, 1). Masters and Johnson reported on the first eleven years of this clinical treatment program in their second book, *Human Sexual Inadequacy*, published in 1970.

THE CONCEPT OF SEX AS A NATURAL FUNCTION

The conceptual starting-point of Masters and Johnson's therapy program is that 'sex is a natural function.' They define a natural function as one that is genetically determined (Masters and Johnson 1976, 250–1). They hold that the body has a genetically determined capacity for sexual response which includes erection of the penis, orgasm, and vaginal lubrication. They point out that since boys can have erections while they are still in the uterus, and girls can have vaginal lubrication and clitoral erections within twenty-four hours of birth, sex is a natural function because there are few opportunities to learn such responses (Masters et al 1985, 217; Irvine 1990a, 90).

Masters and Johnson, however, do not always hold consistently to the idea that sex is a natural function. While they primarily believe that human sexual functioning is natural and pre-social, they sometimes admit that sexual arousal can be taught and thus presumably learned rather than being a natural given. In cases where human sexual functioning is not 'naturally given,' for example, in people experiencing lifelong sexual dysfunctions, Masters et al (1985, 513) claim that 'removing the obstacles to natural functioning is not enough' and that 'teaching' is needed to help these people sexually respond. Although, presumably, some of these lifelong sexual dysfunctions might be immutable were they not subject to therapeutic intervention, it is clear that Masters and his colleagues do not consider these former conditions to be natural. Instead, they think of their own intervention as 'natural' because it facilitates 'appropriate' sexual response. In their discussion of this issue, Masters and his colleagues recognise that sexual functioning is affected by learning but they are less able to see how their ideas about what is natural have been socially constructed (Morrow 1994, 24).

The idea that sex is a natural function may reduce sex to biology, but Irvine (1990a, 90) points out that for Masters and Johnson this is essentially a liberating idea. This is because no matter what the cultural prohibitions and restrictions on sexual expression, Masters and Johnson believe that everybody has a natural sexuality inside of them which can be liberated by the right advice and techniques. This belief was crucial to the development of their sex therapy program. They had a much better chance of marketing their therapy to consumers if they could present a view of 'sex as simple, natural and responsive to technical intervention, not overgrown with thorny social relations' (Irvine 1990a, 91).

THE AETIOLOGY OF SEXUAL DYSFUNCTION

Masters and Johnson believe that when a person's natural sexual function is disrupted or blocked then sexual dysfunctions will occur. In their view, 'Sociocultural deprivation and ignorance of sexual physiology rather than psychiatric or medical illness constitute the etiologic background for most sexual dysfunction' (Masters and Johnson 1970, 21). Davison and Neale (1994, 372–3) have argued that Masters and Johnson (1970) understood the aetiology of sexual dysfunction in terms of a two-tiered model of *current* and *historical* causes. Current causes of sexual dysfunction include what Masters and Johnson call 'fears of performance' and the adoption of a 'spectator role.' Masters and Johnson maintain that if people fear that they cannot sexually perform — such as by developing an erection or having an orgasm — then this fear may become a self-fulfilling prophecy that disrupts their natural sexual response. They state that:

> *fear of inadequacy is the greatest known deterrent to effective sexual functioning, simply because it so completely distracts the fearful individual from his or her natural responsivity by blocking reception of sexual stimuli either created by or reflected from the sexual partner.*
> (Masters and Johnson 1970, 12–13; emphasis in original)

Masters and Johnson also believe that fear of sexual performance might lead to the adoption of a spectator role. This is where individuals mentally disassociate themselves from involvement in sexual activity in order to scrutinise and evaluate their own performances. Masters and Johnson see the adoption of a spectator role as a further inhibition of sexual response (Masters et al 1985, 496–7).

Davison and Neale (1994, 373) point out that Masters and Johnson (1970) believe that the current causes of sexual dysfunction — performance fears and the adoption of a spectator role — may themselves be induced by one of a number of historical antecedents. These antecedents include: 'religious orthodoxy' where individuals have internalised negative religious attitudes to sexual activity; 'psychic trauma' where patients' fear of sexual contact is the result of a frightening or humiliating sexual experience; 'homosexuality' which affects an individual's ability to engage in heterosexual sex; 'negative experiences with counselling' where inadequate or inappropriate advice from professional counsellors results in the causation or exacerbation of sexual dysfunction; 'excessive alcohol intake' which impairs male erectile capacity, and can engender subsequent performance fears which sustain the dysfunction; 'biological causes' including congenital defects, disease, injury, and the effects of drugs, such as tranquillizers; and 'cultural factors', such as the sexual 'double standard', which allows males greater freedom of sexual expression than females (Davison and Neale 1994, 373–4; Masters and Johnson 1970).

Irvine (1990a, 197) argues that one of the main problems with Masters and Johnson's (1970) discussion of the aetiology of sexual dysfunction is that they do not provide an adequate analysis of gender inequality and power in heterosexual relationships. When Masters and Johnson consider gender inequality they tend to sympathise with men who they believe have been unfairly assigned the major cultural responsibility for sexual interaction. Masters and Johnson (1970, 87) think that 'natural sexual interaction' has been impaired by the cultural misconception that men are supposed to be sexual experts who can infallibly divine women's precise sexual needs.

By contrast, Masters and Johnson rarely criticise gender inequalities which disadvantage women. They tend to assume that women and men are equals or that women's 'greater sexual capacity' somehow cancels out their social oppression (Irvine 1990a, 197). They even suggest, at one point, that women's 'greater sexual capacity' has been suppressed because this is functional for the wider society. They say, for example, that a woman's 'significantly greater susceptibility to negatively based psychosocial influences may imply the existence of a natural state of psycho-sexual-social balance between the sexes that has been culturally established to neutralize woman's biophysical superiority' (Masters and Johnson 1970, 219–220).

Masters and Johnson (1970) show little interest in social structural inequalities which might affect women's ability to negotiate safe and pleasurable sexual activity with men. They also appear to have little concern about the way in which women's sexual problems might result from socialisation experiences in a culture that often denies, discourages or devalues female sexuality (Irvine 1990a, 196–7). They seem more interested in the way 'an individual woman internalizes the prevailing psychosocial influence' because they believe this will affect whether or not her sexual value system reinforces 'her natural capacity to function sexually' (Masters and Johnson 1970, 219).

Another problem with Masters and Johnson's (1970) discussion of aetiology concerns the issue of homosexuality. Masters and Johnson regard a 'homophile orientation' as an obstacle to 'natural' heterosexual functioning which can cause erectile dysfunction and ejaculatory incompetence in men, and orgasmic dysfunction and vaginismus in women. Masters and Johnson's treatment program aims to remove these 'obstacles' so that 'satisfactory' heterosexual intercourse can be accomplished. By contrast, they did not develop any therapy programs which enabled heterosexuals to voluntarily convert to homosexuality. This asymmetry reveals the implicit way in which Masters and Johnson regarded heterosexuality as normative and superior to homosexuality (Irvine 1990a, 253).

Masters and Johnson's (1970) discussion of homosexuality as a cause of heterosexual dysfunction also fails to come to grips with issues of power and inequality. They generally fail to understand the way in which the 'personal troubles' of sexually dysfunctional individuals can be connected to 'public issues' of heterosexism and homophobia in the wider society (Mills 1970, ch.1). Masters and Johnson were aware that some homosexual individuals took refuge in heterosexual marriages to escape oppression, and to obtain financial security, social status and public respectability. They also knew that many of these individuals continued to desire same-sex partners and sometimes engaged in extra-marital sex with them. Masters and Johnson realised that in these circumstances it was not surprising that individuals with little or no desire for 'opposite-sex' spouses might develop sexual dysfunctions when they had marital sex. Yet Masters and Johnson tended to pathologise same-sex sexual orientation and to seek its removal through therapy. They preferred this approach over analysing or challenging the oppressive social circumstances which contributed to the predicaments and 'personal troubles' of their patients.

THE GOAL OF SEX THERAPY

The immediate goal of Masters and Johnson's (1970) sex therapy is to reduce or eliminate the causes of sexual dysfunctions — specifically, fears of performance and the spectator role — in order to return sex to its 'natural context.' Unfortunately, they do not actually define what they mean by 'natural context.' Irvine (1990a, 195) presumes that it is 'the state of pure physiological response unencumbered by social or psychological variables.' If this is what Masters and Johnson (1970) mean then it is highly problematic. Szasz (1981, 45–6) points out that no culture accepts sex as a natural function. All societies have prescriptions and proscriptions concerning sex. He agrees that human beings generally have inborn sexual capacities, such as for orgasm, but rightly argues that people nevertheless learn how to think, feel and engage in 'sexual' activities within a wider society. When sexual capacity is understood, activated and experienced within a psychosocial context then Masters and Johnson's goal of returning sex to its natural context seems misconceived and unattainable.

In practice, however, Masters and Johnson (1970) settled for the more modest goal of enabling couples to 'satisfactorily' perform penis in vagina intercourse. They believed, without providing empirical evidence, that sexual dysfunctions were the main cause of divorce in U.S. society and that if these dysfunctions could be cured then marriages would be saved. Their overriding therapeutic goal was to prevent divorce and family break down. This is reflected in their basic therapeutic premise that 'although both husband and wife in a sexually dysfunctional marriage are treated, the marital relationship is considered as the patient' (Masters and Johnson 1970, 3).

DISTINCTIVE ASPECTS OF MASTERS AND JOHNSON'S THERAPEUTIC APPROACH

Masters and Johnson's (1970) therapeutic approach has a number of distinctive elements. Firstly, with some exceptions, Masters and Johnson only accepted couples for treatment. They primarily worked with couples because they believed there are no uninvolved partners in marriages containing sexual inadequacy (Masters and Johnson 1970, 2). They do not necessarily believe that a partner causes the other person's sexual dysfunction, only that the partner and the relationship are affected by it. The strategy of treating couples was also adopted because it was believed to give therapists a better understanding of the couple's problem and an opportunity to elicit 'the co-operation and understanding of both partners in overcoming the distress' (Masters et al 1985, 511).

Masters and Johnson (1970, 146–7) were aware that their preference for treating couples could be seen as discrimination against single people. They decided to overcome this problem by accepting some single people for treatment but treating them as part of a couple. Single people were allowed to have 'replacement partners' accompany them for treatment. These 'replacement partners' were not married to the patients but had ongoing sexual relationships with them. Thirteen men and three women brought replacement partners with them to therapy.

A further problem for Masters and Johnson (1970, 147–8) was how to provide partners for single people who were not involved in ongoing sexual relationships. They decided to solve this problem by providing 'partner surrogates' for single male patients without partners. 'The specific function of the partner surrogate is to approximate insofar as possible the role of a supportive, interested, co-operative wife' (Masters and Johnson 1970, 150). Partner surrogates were paid for their 'wifely' duties which included having sex with the male patients. Surrogates were provided to forty-one single men from a group of thirteen women recruited by Masters and Johnson.

Szasz (1981, 60) has questioned whether there is a difference between clients paying prostitutes for sexual services and patients paying partner surrogates for sexual services. He points out that the patients, surrogates, therapists and those who referred patients to Masters and Johnson's clinic might all have committed offences under laws relating to prostitution. Masters and Johnson were never prosecuted, however, and Szasz (1981, 60) suggests that the medical orientation of their program might have helped to protect them.

Masters and Johnson (1970, 155) did not provide male partner surrogates to single female patients without partners. They were aware that they could be accused of a sexual double standard here. However, they said their clinical decision was based on patients' existing value systems and that these were different for men and women.

A man places primary valuation on his capacity for effective sexual function.... His sexual effectiveness fulfills the requirement of procreation and is honoured with society's approval.... Woman, on the other hand, does not have a similar sexual heritage.... Socioculturally induced requirements are usually reflected by woman's need for a relatively meaningful relationship which can provide her with 'permission' to value her own sexual function. It is the extreme difficulty of meeting this requirement in a brief, two-week period which influenced Foundation policy to deny the incorporation of the male partner surrogate into treatment concepts.... (Masters and Johnson 1970, 155–6)

Masters and Johnson's (1970) attempt to justify their clinical position is based on a problematic essentialist view of male and female sexuality. It is essentialist because of the way in which they see all men as having a common sexual value system which is different from the sexual value system shared by all women. This essentialism is evident even though Masters and Johnson are discussing sociocultural rather than biological aspects of sexuality. Furthermore, their attempt to justify a double standard in their clinical treatment is not convincing. They have basically admitted that 'because a double standard exists in the construction of male and female sexuality....they should continue it because it facilitates treatment' (Jeffreys 1990, 139). Masters and Johnson stopped using female partner surrogates in 1972 after they settled out of court with a man who sued them for prostituting his wife (Wolfe 1978, 496; Heidenry 1997, 168–9).

A second distinctive aspect of Masters and Johnson's (1970) therapy program is that they mirrored the male/female patient couple with a male and female therapist who worked together as part of a dual-sex therapy team. Masters and Johnson (1970, 4–8) claimed that the dual-sex therapy team has a number of advantages over a single therapist. Firstly, it provides each spouse with a 'friend in court' and same sex interpreter who can support and explain her or his views during therapy. Secondly, it avoids a 'two-to-one situation' where the therapist and one spouse 'gang up' against the other spouse. Thirdly, it reduces biases in patient communication with the therapists because patients know they are being monitored by a same sex therapist. Fourthly, it lessens the probability that patients and therapists will become emotionally or sexually involved with each other. If a patient begins showing too much interest in a therapist, then the other therapist can intervene to discourage that interest.

There are, however, a number of problems with Masters and Johnson's (1970) dual-sex therapy approach. Firstly, their concept of dual-sex therapy rests on their claim that male and female patients can only be fully understood by a therapist of the same gender. They say that this claim is unequivocally supported by 'controlled laboratory experimentation in human sexual physiology' (Masters and Johnson 1970, 4). Yet they provide no details of this 'controlled laboratory experimentation' and their claim runs counter to the main finding of their physiological research that males and females are more sexually similar than different (Hogan 1978, 77). It also runs counter to their belief that men and women can better understand each other because they are sexually similar. While Irvine (1990a, 80) believes dual-sex therapy is an 'ideological advance for women' because it moves beyond a single male therapist, other therapists believe that cotherapy is unnecessary and that single 'therapists can be trained to understand the sexuality of opposite-sexed patients' (Hogan 1978, 77).

In his review of cotherapy, Bancroft (1989, 482) agrees with Masters and Johnson that dual-sex therapy reduces the probability that two people will 'gang up' against one. However, he goes on to say that with dual-sex therapy, 'it is not difficult to end up with three against one!' (Bancroft 1989, 482).

Finally, there is little, if any, evidence that dual-sex therapy is any more effective than treatment provided by a single therapist (Hawton 1985, 209–10). However, 'two therapists are twice as expensive as one' and cotherapy has been dropped by most therapists because it reduces access to treatment for lower-income couples (Bancroft 1989, 483; Irvine 1990a, 84).

A third distinctive aspect of Masters and Johnson's (1970) sex therapy program is that they prefer the cotherapists to come from different academic backgrounds, such as from medicine and psychology. The reason for this preference is that the different expertise of the cotherapists can then be combined to improve patient assessment and treatment. Masters and Johnson believe it is particularly important to have a physician as one of the therapists in order to 'identify organic conditions that might require medical or surgical treatment instead of sex therapy' (Masters et al 1985, 511). They complain that, in the past, many psychiatrists did not physically examine patients for fear of eliciting 'unwanted sexual feelings' that could vitiate the treatment relationship (Masters et al 1985, 511).

Finally, in contrast to the long-term nature of many psychoanalytic treatment regimes, Masters and Johnson offered a rapid and intensive program of sex therapy to their patients. Approximately 90% of Masters and Johnson's (1970) patients travelled to their clinic from outside the St. Louis area. These patients stayed in nearby accommodation and were treated on a daily basis at the clinic for two weeks. While in St. Louis, the patients were asked to free themselves from their normal work, family and social commitments so that they could concentrate on improving their relationships (Masters and Johnson 1970, 17–18). Couples who lived in the St. Louis area were seen for three weeks in therapy because it was more difficult for them to isolate themselves from family and business demands (Masters and Johnson 1970, 19–20).

Masters and Johnson's rationale for the two weeks of treatment and social isolation was that couples' 'natural sexual energy' was likely to re-emerge if the cares and concerns of their everyday lives were set aside (Irvine

1990a, 196). Irvine (1990a, 196) points out, however, that the 'problem is that this approach dismisses the extent to which culture, or the workaday world, not only shapes but is an integral part of our own sexuality.' In other words, if the normal patterns of daily life are implicated in the onset or maintenance of sexual dysfunctions or other sexual problems then this is probably what couples will be returning to once they have finished their sojourn in St. Louis. Trying to change only the couple, while leaving the wider circumstances of their lives unchanged, would seem to be a fairly limited therapeutic strategy.

THE NATURE OF MASTERS AND JOHNSON'S SEX THERAPY

Masters and Johnson (1970, 352) stressed that 'The Foundation's therapeutic program for relief of sexual dysfunction is fundamentally a process of marital-unit education with concomitant dissipation of misconception, misinformation, and taboo.' The therapy itself basically consists of giving patients information about sexual anatomy and physiology; advice about effective techniques of sexual stimulation; permission to engage in and enjoy sexual activity; mutual touching exercises to de-emphasise goal-oriented sex; and specific behavioural techniques, such as directed masturbation, for treating particular types of dysfunction, such as female anorgasmia (Masters and Johnson 1970).

THE THERAPY FORMAT

The first four days of the therapy program are basically the same for all patients regardless of their particular sexual dysfunctions. On the first day, the therapists meet the patient couple and explain what will happen over the next four days of the program. At the end of this meeting, the couple is asked not to have intercourse or engage in any other sexual activity until advised by the therapists. This is designed to remove any sexual performance pressure on the couple. After this meeting, the patients are separated and each provides a detailed sociosexual history to the same gender therapist (Masters and Johnson 1970, 30–2). 'History-taking certainly must provide information sufficient to define the character (etiological background, symptom onset, severity and duration, psychosocial affect) of the presenting sexual dysfunction' (Masters and Johnson 1970, 24–5). In order to provide this information, the history-taking focuses on a range of issues including the sexual problems of the couple, the nature of their present marriage, life cycle influences on individual sexual development, sexual feelings, attitudes, experiences and expectations, perception of self and 'awareness of and response to sensory stimuli' (Masters and Johnson

1970, 34–51). Therapists pay particular attention to understanding an individual's 'sexual value system' (what the individual believes is sexually acceptable or unacceptable). This is because Masters and Johnson believe that sexual functioning can be inhibited by the 'wrong' values and attitudes about sexuality. Consequently, a sexual value system might have to be changed before 'normal' sexual functioning can be restored.

On day two of the program, a second history is taken from each spouse but this time on a cross-gender basis: the male therapist interviews the wife and the female therapist interviews the husband. The second interview focuses on any relevant issues omitted in the first interview, any material which is unclear, prejudiced or in need of further exploration (Masters and Johnson 1970, 53–5).

On day three, the spouses provide a medical history, have a physical examination and diagnostic laboratory tests. The therapists and couple then meet in a 'roundtable' discussion. The therapists sum up their findings from the history-taking sessions and physical examinations. They give an explanation of the probable causes of the couple's sexual problem(s) and an estimation of the chances of successful treatment. The couple is invited to correct any factual errors and comment on the therapists' views. The therapists usually discuss the idea that a sexual problem is a problem of the relationship rather than of just one partner; that sex is a natural function; that fears of performance and the adoption of a spectator role are main causes of sexual dysfunctions; and that communication skills are important in resolving the problem (Masters and Johnson 1970, 60–7; Masters et al 1985, 514).

After the roundtable discussion, the therapists usually suggest that the couple tries 'sensate focus' (mutual touching) exercises in the privacy of their own homes or hotel rooms (Masters and Johnson 1970, 71). Masters and Johnson (1970, 76–7) explain that:

> Sensate Focus, the dimension of touch was chosen to provide the sensory experience most easily and appropriately available to marital partners as a medium for physical exchange in reconstituting natural responsivity to sexual stimuli.... These 'exercises' are designed to free sexually dysfunctional individuals from inhibitions that deprive them of an opportunity to respond naturally to sensory experience.... Sensory awareness and its communication to another person can be extremely difficult for those who have not had the opportunity to develop sensate orientation gradually, under circumstances in which the experience was valued and encouraged, or at least not negated.... The educational process, as initiated in therapy by the sensate 'exercises,' permits gradual modification of negative reactions to sensory stimuli so that learning occurs through return from positive experience.

When the sensate focus exercises begin, the couple has two sessions in which each person takes a turn touching the naked body of her or his partner. They are told, however, not to touch the genitals or the female breasts. The person doing the touching is able to caress and explore the other person's body without trying to provoke a sexual response. The person being touched tries to relax and enjoy the sensory experience. The passive partner is not required to sexually respond and is responsible for telling the active partner if any of the touching is uncomfortable. When both partners feel ready, they can change places and repeat the experience (Masters and Johnson 1970, 71–5).

On day four, the therapists and couple meet to discuss the previous day's sensate focus exercises. The therapists are interested in the husband's and wife's reactions and whether they were able to give and receive pleasure without the pressure of a goal-oriented performance. If all goes well, the therapists instruct the couple to try sensate exploration twice more before the next therapy session on day five. The exercises are to proceed as before but with two additional instructions. Firstly, the touching can now be extended to include the genitals and the female breasts. The therapists make sure during the discussion that the husband and wife understand genital anatomy. The couple are told, however, that they should not try to induce orgasm through their genital touching. Secondly, the person being touched is told to put her/his hand on top of the touching partner's hand in order to indicate personal preferences in the type of touching required. This facilitates the development of the partners' non-verbal communication skills (Masters and Johnson 1970, 85–91). Masters and Johnson (1970, 89) state that 'Any level of sexual responsivity spontaneously developing in this unpressured, nonperformance-oriented situation, is, of course, the ultimate purpose of the exercises.' The couple is also told to repeat the sensate focus exercises on every subsequent day of the therapy program so that they become a normal part of their sexual interaction (Masters and Johnson 1970, 86).

Following Masters and Johnson's (1970) work, many therapists believed sensate focus to be an important therapeutic tool and an essential component of sex therapy (Tiefer 1995, 137). LoPiccolo (1992, 188–9) points out, however, that sensate focus often fails to produce erections in contemporary patients seeking help for erectile dysfunction. He argues that one of the reasons for this is that sensate focus is, in a sense, a paradoxical form of treatment. The paradox is that people are both expected and not expected to sexually respond during sensate focus (Davison and Neale 1994, 379). Therapists encourage patients to relax and enjoy sensate focus without feeling pressured to produce a sexual response. However, the therapists also expect that the elimination of performance anxiety will enable patients to sexually respond. This is the ultimate purpose of sensate focus. LoPiccolo

(1992, 189) argues that if patients are aware of this underlying purpose then instead of suffering from performance anxiety they may instead suffer from 'metaperformance anxiety.' One of LoPiccolo's patients explains the nature of 'metaperformance anxiety' in this way:

> I found myself lying there, thinking, 'I'm now free of pressure to perform. I'm not supposed to get an erection, and we're not allowed to have intercourse even if I do get one. So now that all the pressure is off, why am I not getting an erection? I'm relaxed, I'm enjoying this, so where's the erection?' (LoPiccolo 1992, 189)

LoPiccolo (1992, 189) argues that sensate focus is only likely to work if patients are unaware of the paradoxical nature of the treatment. This itself is becoming less likely due to increasing media attention to sex therapy techniques. Patients who are aware of the paradox, on the other hand, are likely to experience metaperformance anxiety 'about why eliminating performance anxiety does not lead to...[sexual response] during sensate focus body massage' (LoPiccolo 1992, 189).

THE TREATMENT OF SPECIFIC DYSFUNCTIONS

On day five of Masters and Johnson's sex therapy program, the patient couple is treated for the specific dysfunction(s) which brought it to therapy. The main features of Masters and Johnson's (1970) treatment model are then supplemented by additional techniques used in the treatment of specific dysfunctions. The treatment of specific dysfunctions is described below.

Premature ejaculation

In the treatment of premature ejaculation, the main aim is to teach the husband how to delay his ejaculation. The wife begins by caressing his genitals until he has an erection. Then she uses the 'squeeze technique.' She places her thumb on the frenulum of the penis and her two fingers on each side of the coronal ridge on the opposite side of the penis. She firmly squeezes her thumb and fingers for about four seconds and then releases. This pressure reduces the man's urge to ejaculate although it is not known why this happens. The squeeze may also cause partial or temporary loss of erection. After fifteen to thirty seconds, the wife again fondles her husband to produce an erection and again squeezes his penis to prevent ejaculation. This exercise can be repeated to produce fifteen to twenty minutes of sexual stimulation without ejaculation (Masters and Johnson 1970, 102–4).

In the next step, the wife straddles her husband and inserts his penis into her vagina. She does not move so that her husband can get used to a feeling of vaginal containment without any urge to ejaculate. Once this is accomplished, the husband is told to thrust his penis just enough to maintain his erection. The squeeze technique is again used if the man feels he is about to ejaculate (Masters and Johnson 1970, 106–8).

When the couple can manage motionless and slow-motion intercourse for fifteen to twenty minutes in the female superior position, they are taught to have intercourse in the side-by-side position. This latter position is said to be the best for maintaining ejaculatory control. The couple is told that when they go home from therapy they should practise the squeeze technique at least once a week for the first six months. Masters and Johnson report that ejaculatory control is usually accomplished in six to twelve months (Masters and Johnson 1970, 108–12).

Ejaculatory incompetence

Treatment for ejaculatory incompetence begins with the wife manually stimulating her husband's penis in the ways he finds most exciting. Her aim is to make him ejaculate. Once she has succeeded, she practises her technique until he can easily ejaculate from her manipulation. In the next step of therapy, the wife masturbates her husband's penis until he is almost ready to ejaculate. She then adopts the female superior position and inserts his penis into her vagina. She continues to move demandingly on his penis until he ejaculates (Masters and Johnson 1970, 129–32). 'After three or four such episodes of rapid intravaginal penetration as the male is ejaculating, confidence in intravaginal ejaculatory performance will have been established' (Masters and Johnson 1970, 132). Finally, the therapists encourage the husband and wife to increase the amount of time his penis is in her vagina before he ejaculates so that she can also have a coital orgasm (Masters and Johnson 1970, 132).

Impotence

The treatment of impotence is also an extension of the sensate focus exercises used to reduce fears of performance and the adoption of a spectator role. When the man begins to have erections during these exercises, the couple is encouraged to experiment with his erectile ability. Masters and Johnson (1970, 206) emphasise that 'the most effective step in the physical aspect of the therapeutic program' is the 'teasing' technique. The wife is advised to tease her husband's penis into erection; cease stimulation so that the erection is lost; and recommence stimulation to produce another erection. She is supposed to repeat this pattern for at least half an hour in a slow and nondemanding way (Masters and Johnson 1970, 206). The teasing technique is designed to overcome the man's fears of losing his erection and being unable to get it back.

When the man can experience erections from the teasing technique, the next step is for the wife to straddle her husband and insert his penis into her vagina (Masters and Johnson 1970, 206). 'This reduces pressures on the man to decide when it is time to insert and removes the potential distraction of his fumbling to "find" the vagina' (Masters et al 1985, 518). This manoeuvre is to be practised until 'erective security develops' (Masters and Johnson 1970, 208).

After this has been accomplished, the next step is for the wife to slowly move up and down on her husband's penis. If he loses his erection, she is to withdraw, manually stimulate his penis to erection, re-lodge it in her vagina and continue the exercise. After several minutes of gentle thrusting, the wife remains still and her husband thrusts slowly to feel the warmth and constriction of her vagina (Masters and Johnson 1970, 209–10).

On subsequent days the couple is encouraged to engage in simultaneous 'pelvic pleasuring' and to enjoy the 'mutuality of their sexual stimulation' (Masters and Johnson 1970, 210). The couple is told not to be concerned about reaching orgasm in these exercises. However, if it occurs it should happen 'involuntarily' and 'naturally' (Masters and Johnson 1970, 210).

Female orgasmic dysfunction

The earlier sensate focus exercises are also used as a basis for treatment of female orgasmic dysfunction. The husband sits up on the bed against the headboard and the wife leans back against him in between his legs. She spreads her legs by crossing them over to the outside of his legs. She also places her hand on top of his to show him how she likes to be touched. Masters and Johnson recommend that the man begins with a light teasing touch over the woman's breasts, belly and thighs, eventually moving to the general area of the clitoris. The woman controls the type of stimulation provided and communicates her preferences to her husband. The partners are discouraged from striving for orgasm. The purpose of the exercise is to allow the woman to enjoy the experience, discover how she likes to be stimulated and to communicate this information to her husband (Masters and Johnson 1970, 300–4).

When the couple reports that the wife has been aroused by the genital touching, the therapists advise the wife to mount her husband and insert his penis into her vagina. She is told to lie still so that she can enjoy the feeling of penile containment. As she feels the need to increase sexual stimulation she can begin some slow controlled pelvic thrusting. After several sessions practising this exercise, the wife may begin to experience vaginal sensation. The husband is then instructed to commence pelvic thrusting in a slow nondemanding way and is guided by his wife's preferences. The therapists emphasise that any spontaneous orgasm which occurs is no cause for alarm and should just be enjoyed (Masters and Johnson 1970, 306–8).

In subsequent therapy, the husband and wife are advised to engage in slow non-demanding intercourse for as long as it is pleasurable. During this intercourse, the partners are encouraged to take two or three breaks from coitus and lie in each other's arms while they rest. After resting they can return to manual sensate pleasuring, then reinsertion of the penis in the vagina, and lying quietly together or with slow pelvic thrusting (Masters and Johnson 1970, 308).

In the final stage of therapy the couple is taught to change from the female superior position to a side-by-side position. The latter position is said to allow the woman to better regulate her own pelvic thrusting and give the man better ejaculatory control. The woman usually achieves an orgasm before the rapid treatment program is over (Masters and Johnson 1970, 310–14).

Vaginismus

In the treatment of vaginismus the therapists firstly explain the condition to the couple using anatomical illustrations. Then the therapist physically examines the woman. The therapist demonstrates the existence of a vaginal spasm to the couple by attempting to insert her or his finger. The husband is also asked to feel the constriction. Once the existence of vaginismus has been demonstrated to the couple they are given a set of different sized dilators which they are supposed to use in private to reduce the spasms. The therapists first advise the woman to manually control her husband's insertion of a small dilator into her vagina. As she becomes more confident of accepting the dilator, she instructs her husband to try progressively larger sizes for insertion. When she can accommodate a large dilator (about the size of an erect penis) she is encouraged to retain it in her vagina for several hours each night. If the dilators are used every day most of the involuntary spasm will be eliminated in three to five days. Occasionally the dilators may be needed prior to intercourse in the first six weeks after treatment but for many patients the spasm can be permanently removed in a few days. Once this occurs, the therapists and the couple discuss the causes of vaginismus (Masters and Johnson 1970, 262–3). Masters and Johnson (1970, 264–5) believe that a combination of physical therapy and sex education is usually sufficient to successfully treat the couple.

THE ORIGINALITY OF MASTERS AND JOHNSON'S SEX THERAPY PROGRAM

Although Masters and colleagues (1985, 21) claimed that *Human Sexual Inadequacy* was 'a landmark book that described a *startlingly new approach* to the treatment of sexual problems', many of their treatment principles and techniques were not original (emphasis added). The impression that their treatment approach was atheoretical and based solely on their empirical work might have been fostered by Masters and Johnson's (1970, 1) claim that 'Current treatment concepts are founded on a combination of

15 years of laboratory experimentation and 11 years of clinical trial and error' (Bancroft 1989, 462). In actual fact, however, their treatment program is largely based on the principles and techniques of behaviour therapy (Wilson 1982, 539). These include:

> the identification of anxiety as the primary cause of dysfunctional behavior; viewing overt symptomatic behavior as the target of change, rather than hypothetical underlying intrapsychic conflicts; changing undesired behaviors through step-by-step successive approximation to the desired end goal; and using active directed behavioral assignments for promoting behavioral change, rather than insight and interpretation. (Leiblum and Pervin 1980, 15–16)

Masters and Johnson did not describe their treatment methods as behaviour therapy, however, and this led some critics to accuse them of plagiarising behaviour therapy techniques (Wilson 1982, 539; Bancroft 1989, 462). Masters et al (1985, 522) later conceded that 'many methods used by Masters and Johnson are very similar to behavioral techniques....'

Even some of the more specific treatment strategies and techniques that Masters and Johnson used were not original. Alfred Kinsey and Albert Ellis had previously written about the importance of clitoral stimulation in female sexual response; the temporary ban on sexual intercourse for patients had been described over 180 years earlier by John Hunter; and the famous squeeze technique for premature ejaculation was reportedly used by prostitutes before Masters and Johnson learned of it and incorporated it into their therapy program (Irvine 1990a, 192; Hunter 1963 [1786]; Heidenry 1997, 30). In *Human Sexual Response*, Masters and Johnson (1966, 10) openly acknowledged that the prostitutes Masters worked with in the early stages of his research on sexual physiology provided them with many techniques which could be directly applied in sex therapy.

Masters and Johnson's treatment program differed from earlier approaches, however, in that it included treatment of a couple by a couple; brief intensive therapy rather than one session a week over months or years; and specific treatment packages for each of the sexual dysfunctions (Zilbergeld and Evans 1980, 29). Most importantly, though, they integrated a variety of existing treatment strategies and techniques into a more comprehensive package that seemed to make sense, and which appealed to many therapists 'working with more conventional behavioural therapy techniques...' (Bancroft 1989, 462).

MASTERS AND JOHNSON'S (1970) CLINICAL TREATMENT RESULTS

In *Human Sexual Inadequacy*, Masters and Johnson (1970) reported their results of treating 790 patients for sexual dysfunctions over an eleven year period from January 1959 to December 1969. This is the 'largest series of treated cases for which outcome has been reported' (Bancroft 1989, 493; Heiman and Meston 1997, 149). Masters and Johnson (1970, 367) regarded 142 patients as treatment failures out of the 790 patients they treated. This is a failure rate of 18% which Masters and Johnson (1970, 367) incorrectly reported as 18.9%. The failure rates for the particular types of sexual dysfunction are listed below:

Primary impotence	40.6%
Secondary impotence	26.2%
Situational orgasmic dysfunction	22.8%
Ejaculatory incompetence	17.6%
Primary orgasmic dysfunction	16.6%
Premature ejaculation	2.2%
Vaginismus	No failures

(Masters and Johnson 1970, 358–60, 367)

There were no significant clinical differences in the failure rates for male and female patients when all types of sexual dysfunction were considered. The failure rate for male patients was 16.9% and the corresponding rate for females was 19.3% (Masters and Johnson 1970, 361).

Masters and Johnson (1970, 361–9) also included data on the 'long term' results of their intensive therapy program. They followed-up patients five years after their initial therapy in order to find out how many had reverted to their earlier patterns of sexual dysfunction. Unfortunately, Masters and Johnson's discussion of how many patients they actually followed-up is confusing and inconsistent. As a result, some readers thought Masters and Johnson followed-up all 790 of their patients (Zilbergeld and Evans 1980, 37); some thought they followed-up only 313 of their patients (Wilson 1982, 539); some thought they followed-up 313 patient couples (Hawton 1985, 201; Bancroft 1989, 494); some thought they followed-up 282 patients (Belliveau and Richter 1971, 227); others that they followed-up 226 patients (Zilbergeld and Evans 1980, 37; Kolodny 1981, 310). The actual number seems to be 226 patients.

Masters and Johnson (1970, 362) treated 313 married and single patients between January 1959 and December 1964. They wanted to follow-up each cohort from these first six years of treatment for five years after treatment. Thus, patients first treated in 1959 would be followed-up in 1964, and patients treated in 1964 would be followed-up in 1969. However, eighty-seven patients were lost to the follow-up program. Fifty-six of these patients were not included in the follow-up because they were initial treatment failures. The other thirty-one patients who were initial treatment successes lost contact with the therapists and were excluded from the follow-up. This left 226 patients as the total number to be followed-up out of the original 313 (Masters and Johnson 1970, 362–4). Eleven years after *Human Sexual Inadequacy* was first published, Robert Kolodny (1981,

310), Associate Director of Training at the Masters and Johnson Institute, confirmed that '5 year follow-up data were presented in *Human Sexual Inadequacy* for 226 out of 313 cases treated between 1959 and 1964....' Masters and Johnson themselves reviewed Kolodny's (1981) paper before it was published so presumably this is the correct figure.

Masters and Johnson (1970, 365) originally stated that these 226 patients were personally interviewed between four-and-a-half to five-and-a-half years after they had completed the two-week therapy program. They then said that 'The remaining eighty-seven individuals [who they previously said were excluded from the follow-up] had their final five-year interviews conducted by telephone' (Masters and Johnson 1970, 365). Furthermore, they said 'It is on the basis of these final interviews that an ultimate decision as to treatment reversal (TR) was established and opportunity taken to describe the reversal rate (RR) percentage for the follow-up population' (Masters and Johnson 1970, 365). Masters and Johnson (1970, 365) seem to suggest in these passages that the eighty-seven previously excluded individuals were now included in the follow-up group. This might explain why some readers thought the total follow-up population was 313 rather than 226 individuals.

Masters and Johnson (1970, 366) created further confusion by presenting their results in a table called 'Five-Year Follow-Up of *313 Marital Units,* 1959–1964' when they had previously pointed out that their original treatment population consisted of '313 *individual* cases of sexual inadequacy' (Masters and Johnson 1970, 362; emphasis added). These 313 individual cases consisted of 301 cases of sexual dysfunction in *215 marital units* (couples) plus sexual dysfunctions in twelve individuals (Masters and Johnson 1970, 362). Despite having confused marital units with individuals, Masters and Johnson then presented the failure rate for 313 marital units over a five year period. There were sixteen failures which gave a failure rate of 5.1%. If the follow-up population was actually 226 individuals, as Masters and Johnson (1970, 362–4) previously indicated, and Kolodny (1981, 310) confirmed, then the failure rate was really 7%.

Masters and Johnson (1970, 367) also reported that their overall failure rate — which was comprised of 158 total failures, (in turn, comprised of 142 initial therapy failures and sixteen failures in follow-up) divided by the total number of patients (790) — was 20%. Kolodny (1981, 311) points out that 'If the reversal rates found in the 5 year follow-up group [1959–1964] were extrapolated to the cases treated between 1965 and 1969, the overall failure rate would be 23% rather than 20%, as it is listed.'

THE IMPACT OF MASTERS AND JOHNSON

Prior to 1970, in the United States, psychoanalysis was the main form of treatment for sexual dysfunctions. Treatment was lengthy and success was uncertain (Pryde 1989, 215). In 1970, however, Masters and Johnson published *Human Sexual Inadequacy*. This book claimed to offer a new way of treating sexual dysfunctions which avoided lengthy treatment and high failure rates.

> With a two-week treatment program and only a 20 percent failure rate, this work was soon to give rise to an entire new profession — sex therapy — with the eventual proliferation of thousands of sex clinics across the country before the end of the decade.... (Masters et al 1985, 21)

Zilbergeld and Evans (1980, 30) point out that it is rare for a new form of treatment to become established as quickly as sex therapy. Masters and Johnson were able to make the new field respectable in only a few years.

> Today there are thousands of sex therapists, two organizations to certify them, and at least two professional journals devoted to their endeavours. Even many traditional therapists use the new methods, or variations of them, in their work or refer patients with sex problems to those who do. (Zilbergeld and Evans 1980, 30)

Leiblum and Pervin (1980, 14–15) argue that there were many factors which contributed to the growth of sex therapy and demand for its services: improving birth control technology in the 1950s helped to produce a shift of emphasis from sexuality for procreation to sexuality for recreation; changing lifestyles and increasing independence for many women provided them with the encouragement to lead more 'liberated' sexual lives; the 'counterculture' of the 1960s challenged authoritarian and repressive restrictions on many forms of human behaviour and valorized spontaneity and sensuality; increasing media coverage of sexual issues 'helped destigmatize discussion of, and fostered interest in sexual satisfaction for all individuals, not just the young and beautiful'; Masters and Johnson's research on human sexual response led many medical schools to offer courses on human sexuality; and graduate students from a variety of disciplines were educated about their work.

Masters and Johnson's (1970) claims about the brevity and effectiveness of their therapy program were also important reasons for its popular reception. Their claims were accepted with little critical scrutiny as people were 'swept away in the tidal wave of excitement and congratulation' which followed the publication of *Human Sexual Inadequacy* (Zilbergeld and Evans 1980, 42). Reviewers hailed *Human Sexual Inadequacy* as a 'landmark,' 'revolutionary' and 'epoch-making.' One reviewer wrote that 'The authors...suggest that human sexual inadequacy could be substantially eliminated in the next 10 years. This is a bold claim; yet in the light of the encouraging programs which the book reports, it may indeed be a justifiable one' (Zilbergeld and Evans 1980, 30).

A reviewer for the *Washington Post* wrote that 'Their results are dramatically convincing.' The review in the *New York Times* described Masters and Johnson's work as 'extraordinary' and 'phenomenal' (Zilbergeld and Evans 1980, 30). 'An air of optimism and enthusiasm prevailed as therapists, counsellors and educators hurried to learn and dispense the Masters and Johnson methods' (Pryde 1989, 215). In April 1970, Masters and Johnson acknowledged that they had already cleared the applications of over 200 dual-sex therapy teams for training (Lehrman 1976, 87).

Zilbergeld and Evans (1980, 42–3) suggest that there were probably five main reasons for the lack of critical scrutiny of Masters and Johnson's (1970) work. Firstly, the widespread acclaim for *Human Sexual Response* helped Masters and Johnson to acquire reputations as rigorous scientists. Their reputations, in turn, seem to have created a 'halo effect' on the reception of *Human Sexual Inadequacy*. Secondly, Masters and Johnson's writing style is taxing, turgid and often imprecise about key details of their research and therapy. This leads many readers to respond to their work in ways which are not conducive to criticism: many readers skim the long, dry, difficult sections of text, and concentrate more on the treatments and outcome statistics which give a more positive picture than is justified; many people 'read between the lines' of the vague passages and supply meanings which are not actually there; and others incorrectly translate ambiguous terms such as 'satisfaction' into more specific terms such as 'orgasm'. 'By supplying the coherence and specificity lacking in the text, readers eliminate some of the grounds for criticism' (Zilbergeld and Evans 1980, 43). Thirdly, Masters and Johnson present themselves in their texts as self-critical researchers. They often confess their inadequacies, mistakes and ignorance. Zilbergeld and Evans (1980, 43) believe that such humility may deter reviewers from fully criticising their work. Alternatively, their self-critical orientation might lead normally critical readers to believe that Masters and Johnson have already identified the main weaknesses in their work. Fourthly, most sexologists are keenly aware of their debt to the 'pioneering' work of Masters and Johnson. They realise that to criticise Masters and Johnson is, in effect, to undermine the very foundation which supports their own work and reputations. Finally, Zilbergeld and Evans (1980, 43) suggest that when *Human Sexual Inadequacy* was published, sexology was still a relatively young field, and its standards for the presentation and publication of research findings were less stringent than in more established disciplines.

Human Sexual Inadequacy did not entirely escape criticism, however. There was initial criticism from psychiatrists and psychoanalysts who were Masters and Johnson's main competitors in the 'sex therapy' market. The sociologist, John Gagnon, for example, points out that a number of psychiatrists were concerned about Masters and Johnson's work because psychiatrists alone were regarded as the experts on sex before Masters and Johnson came along. He says:

It was threatening enough to the profession when Masters and Johnson set about with their original research into the nature of sexual response. But now that they have gone into therapy, many traditional therapists will be as jittery as the plumbers union is when faced with a possible incursion of blacks into their ranks. (Cadden 1978, 488)

Irvine (1990a, 194–5) argues that Masters and Johnson's (1970) sex therapy program had a number of marketing advantages over traditional psychotherapy. Firstly, 'the very existence of sex therapy programs validated people's hopes and desires for better sex' (Irvine 1990a, 194). Many people realised that it was now legitimate to seek 'professional' help to have an orgasm or maintain an erection rather than just to hope that those experiences might occur as by-products of lengthy psychoanalysis. Secondly, Masters and Johnson's treatment was brief, and aimed to remove the dysfunction rather than any deep psychological causes which might have produced it. Masters and Johnson believed that sexual dysfunctions were learned inhibitions in the natural cycle of human sexual response which could be modified by new learning. This distinguished their treatment approach from psychoanalysis which viewed sexual dysfunctions as symptoms of largely unconscious processes which originated in early childhood. Finally, Masters and Johnson's enthusiastic claim of excellent treatment results was probably the major selling point of their program. It provided a stark contrast to the poor record of their chief competitors (Zilbergeld and Kilmann 1984, 319).

Confronted with Masters and Johnson's (1970) challenge to their authority and business, psychiatrists and psychoanalysts responded in a number of ways. Some chose to ignore Masters and Johnson and continued to supply their own forms of therapy (Irvine 1990a, 77). Some accepted Masters and Johnson's claims of therapeutic success and withdrew from the 'sex therapy' market back to the 'identity therapy' market (Bejin 1986a, 200). Some criticised Masters and Johnson and continued to extol the virtues of psychoanalysis (Kolodny 2001, 275). Natalie Shainess, for example, discussed Masters and Johnson's sex therapy as a form of 'coaching that reduces one partner to a push-button operator' (Cadden 1978, 487). She was also concerned that it 'papered over' symptoms which would reappear because the underlying deep causes of the dysfunctions had not been treated (Cadden 1978, 487). Many other psychiatrists, however, eventually incorporated some of Masters and Johnson's treatment principles and techniques into their own therapeutic repertoires (Rosen 1977). One psychoanalyst, Helen Kaplan (1978), even produced a synthesis between psychoanalysis and Masters and Johnson's (1970) therapeutic approach to produce what she called the 'new sex therapy.'

It was not until 1980, however, that the first serious challenge to Masters and Johnson's (1970) claims was published. This was Zilbergeld and

Evans's (1980) critique of Masters and Johnson's claims about their therapy's effectiveness.

THE EFFECTIVENESS OF MASTERS AND JOHNSON'S (1970) SEX THERAPY

Irvine (1990a, 199) points out that the marketing of sex therapy depends heavily on its claims of providing effective treatment for sexual dysfunctions. Masters and Johnson's (1970) report of remarkable treatment results from their brief, intensive therapy program was the most important factor in raising the profile and popularity of sex therapy. Their report provided the basis for claims of sex therapy's effectiveness for many years (Zilbergeld and Evans 1980, 29, 33). Yet while Masters and Johnson's claims were generally accepted, and 'an astounding five thousand sex-therapy clinics sprouted up in the wake of *HSI [Human Sexual Inadequacy]*' (Heidenry 1997, 172), few controlled outcome studies were conducted to evaluate the effectiveness of sex therapy (Heiman and Meston 1997). Hogan (1978, 58) pointed out, for example, that the 'majority of papers published on the treatment of sexual dysfunctions merely report single case studies or series of case studies.'

At the time *Human Sexual Inadequacy* was published, Masters and Johnson (1970, 351) emphasised that 'reported successes in any new form of clinical treatment have had only one impeccable judgmental yardstick: are the reported successes reproducible in other geographical areas, by independent clinical treatment centres, following outlined techniques of therapy?' They accepted that this was the clinical yardstick which could 'be applied without reservation' to their own therapeutic program (Masters and Johnson 1970, 352). Seven years later, Sallie Schumacher reviewed the effectiveness of sex therapy. She noted that because Masters and Johnson's 'approach is not practical for most patients and sometimes not appropriate..., there are no reports in the literature on the effectiveness of this particular treatment method other than that presented by Masters and Johnson' (Schumacher 1977, 142).

Zilbergeld and Evans (1980, 30) began to question Masters and Johnson's (1970) treatment results when they noticed that they, and other sex therapists, were not able to match Masters and Johnson's low rates of treatment failure. Evans wanted to replicate Masters and Johnson's study with a college population but was unable to do so because vital information was missing from *Human Sexual Inadequacy*. Zilbergeld and Evans (1980, 33) wrote:

> Our analysis forces us to conclude that Masters and Johnson have not provided the information necessary for either intelligent interpretation or replication. There are huge gaps in their presentation. Essential information about the duration of therapy, the criteria and measures

used to assess treatment effects initially and on follow-up, and the characteristics of the patient population either are not given or are presented in confusing ways. And some findings are reported in a misleading manner.

Zilbergeld and Evans (1980) outlined in detail the major methodological and reporting problems with Masters and Johnson's (1970) treatment outcome research. Firstly, Masters and Johnson (1970, 351) reported their outcomes in terms of failure rates because they argued that therapists and patients could more easily agree on what was a failure rather than on what was a success. They defined initial failure 'as indication that the two-week rapid-treatment phase has failed to initiate reversal of the basic symptomatology of sexual dysfunction for which the unit [couple] was referred to the Foundation' (Masters and Johnson 1970, 352–3). However, Masters and Johnson did not define what the words 'initiating reversal' actually meant. They might mean, for example, that an anorgasmic woman feels less guilty about sex, is less performance oriented, enjoys sex more or reaches orgasm through masturbation or intercourse. But it is not clear 'which, if any, of these changes [would] lead Masters and Johnson to classify an anorgasmic woman as a nonfailure' (Zilbergeld and Evans 1980, 33). Moreover, treatment failure rates will vary depending on how success or failure is defined. It is generally much easier, for example, for an anorgasmic woman to learn to have orgasms through masturbation than through her partner's manual or oral stimulation, or through intercourse. Masters and Johnson (1970), however, did not provide 'outcome criteria for any of the female dysfunctions' (Zilbergeld and Evans 1980, 33). They later claimed this was because they wrote *Human Sexual Inadequacy* in a hurry and inadvertently omitted the outcome criteria (Wolinsky 1983, 2).

In the case of male dysfunctions, the outcome criteria seemed to be more specific but there were still unresolved problems. For example, Masters and Johnson (1970, 157) diagnosed secondary impotence when 'an individual male's rate of failure at successful coital connection approaches 25 percent of his opportunities....' However, they did not say what 'successful coital connection' meant or whether it referred, for example, to the firmness or duration of the man's erection or the subjective satisfaction of the man or his partner. Similarly, they did not say what they meant by 'approaches 25 percent.' If a man after therapy is unsuccessful in 20% of his coital encounters, would Masters and Johnson regard him as a failure or nonfailure? (Zilbergeld and Evans 1980, 34).

Furthermore, Masters and Johnson (1970) did not describe or list their evaluation measures. This meant there was no information on whether patients evaluated their own progress, such as by filling in questionnaires. The therapists apparently made the final evaluation but there was no information on what happened if the therapists, or the therapists and the patients disagreed (Zilbergeld and Evans 1980, 34).

The second problem with Masters and Johnson's (1970) report concerned the issue of nonfailure. They did not define 'nonfailure' or provide a way to assess the extent of therapeutic improvement in the 80% of patients lumped together in the nonfailure category. Most people probably assumed when reading *Human Sexual Inadequacy* that a 20% failure rate implied an 80% success rate. Masters and Johnson denied this, however, and their comments suggested that not all nonfailures could be regarded as successes. Their category of nonfailure appeared to include a variety of patients with treatment outcomes ranging from slight improvement to complete resolution of their problems. Because Masters and Johnson did not define nonfailure or use more discriminating categories for their outcome assessment — such as 'problem resolved,' 'marked improvement,' 'no change,' and 'deterioration' — it was impossible to tell how many patients fell into each category. It was also impossible to compare Masters and Johnson's treatment outcomes with the outcomes of other therapists who did use such categories (Zilbergeld and Evans 1980, 34).

The third problem was that Masters and Johnson (1970) provided insufficient data for other clinicians and researchers to tell how they selected or rejected patients for therapy. Masters and Johnson did not say how many applicants they rejected. Nor did they indicate how many patients dropped out of therapy or whether any 'drop-outs' were regarded as failures. It is very difficult for other therapists to try and replicate Masters and Johnson's research if such basic information about their patient sample is missing (Zilbergeld and Evans 1980, 34–5).

The fourth problem concerned Masters and Johnson's (1970) follow-up data. The presentation of their data was confusing and many reviewers have been mistaken about just how many patients Masters and Johnson actually included in their follow-up study. In addition, Masters and Johnson reported a 'relapse rate of 7 percent [which] is probably the lowest ever reported for any treatment with such a long follow-up' (Zilbergeld and Evans 1980, 37). Yet almost nothing is known about the follow-up study. There is no information even on whether patients were asked a standard set of questions or what specific questions they were asked (Zilbergeld and Evans 1980, 38).

It is also difficult to determine whether Masters and Johnson's (1970) relapse rate was lower than that of other therapists because Masters and Johnson's treatment was superior or because their criteria of patient relapse were less stringent. In terms of treatment quality, Masters and Johnson provided very little information about how they prepared patients for the period following intensive therapy. Nor did they give much information about the therapists' follow-up telephone calls which might have assisted patients in maintaining any therapeutic gains. Without this information the quality of their treatment could not be effectively evaluated (Zilbergeld and Evans 1980, 38).

Another possible explanation of Masters and Johnson's (1970) low relapse rate is that they used less stringent criteria of relapse than other therapists. Masters and Johnson claimed their criteria were stringent. They said that if patients are to be classified as nonfailures then they must continue to improve after their intensive therapy finishes. However, Zilbergeld and Evans (1980, 38) argue that this claim of stringency is more a matter of rhetoric than reality. They point out, for example, that when twenty-three men who were treated for premature ejaculation developed secondary impotence just prior to, or shortly after, the end of the two week therapy program, Masters and Johnson excluded them from the reported relapse rates.

The fifth problem with Masters and Johnson's (1970) research was that they appeared to understate the total amount of time in which their patients received therapy. Masters and Johnson referred to a two-week therapy program for visitors to St. Louis (and three weeks for St. Louis residents) but they did not say how many hours of therapy these patients received. In addition to regular phone calls between the therapists and patients after intensive therapy, patients were also instructed to call their therapists if any sexual problems occurred. Masters and Johnson apparently did not regard these calls as treatment. Zilbergeld and Evans (1980, 38), however, argued that these calls may have lasted some time and involved reassurance and advice which helped couples to resolve their sexual problems. In short, the phone calls may have been a form of treatment. Masters and Johnson, however, did not provide information on the frequency, duration or content of phone calls after the intensive therapy stage so the overall duration of their therapy was not known. Zilbergeld and Evans (1980, 38) suggest that in cases where monthly phone calls of thirty minutes duration occurred over a few years the actual duration of Masters and Johnson's therapy would have been substantially greater than they have acknowledged. The lack of information about the actual duration of their therapy made it impossible to say 'whether Masters and Johnson's therapy is longer, shorter, or the same length as the sex therapy offered by others' (Zilbergeld and Evans 1980, 40).

The final problem with Masters and Johnson's (1970) research concerned the harmful effects of sex therapy. Masters and Johnson acknowledged that therapeutic shortcomings and mistakes precipitated at least two divorces among couples that they treated but they did not indicate that they examined any other ways in which their therapy might have harmed patients. Nor did they follow-up patients who were initial therapy failures. This was the group most likely to experience negative effects from therapy and both of the aforementioned divorced couples came from this group (Zilbergeld and Evans 1980, 40).

As mentioned previously, Masters and Johnson (1970) did not have a treatment outcome category of 'deterioration.' Instead, they used a broad category of 'failure' which included patients who were 'failures' in different senses of the word. Some patients were 'failures' with valued ongoing relationships whose sexual dysfunctions were not 'cured.' Other patients were regarded as 'failures' because they became distraught during therapy and eventually terminated their relationships. Zilbergeld and Evans (1980, 40) argue that lumping these different cases together in a common category of failure serves to hide any harm caused by the therapy. In conclusion, Zilbergeld and Evans (1980, 29–30) stated that:

> Masters and Johnson's research is so flawed by methodological errors and slipshod reporting that it fails to meet customary standards — and their own — for evaluation research.... From reading what they write, it is impossible to tell what the results were. Because of this, the effectiveness of sex therapy — widely assumed to be high since the advent of Masters and Johnson — is thrown into question.

Masters and Johnson declined to respond to Zilbergeld and Evans' (1980) critique because it was published in a 'popular forum' (*Psychology Today*) and they kept silent in the following months. The critique went largely unnoticed and many therapists continued to cite Masters and Johnson's (1970) treatment outcome statistics as evidence of sex therapy's effectiveness (Zilbergeld and Evans 1980, 33; Heidenry 1997, 285).

In 1981, Robert Kolodny, Associate Director and Director of Training at the Masters and Johnson Institute, replied to a number of Zilbergeld and Evans' (1980) questions and criticisms. He revealed that in Masters and Johnson's (1970) therapy program the therapists were the only ones to evaluate the patients' treatment outcomes. If the therapists disagreed, they would consult with one of the directors of the Foundation to make a judgement. The sole criterion used to evaluate treatment outcome was the patient's sexual functioning not his or her attitudinal change or subjective sexual satisfaction. The category of treatment 'failure' included cases that showed more or less improvement in sexual functioning as well as cases that showed no improvement at all. The category of 'nonfailure' 'included only cases that were unequivocal successes in the reversal of sexual symptomatology' (Kolodny 1981, 303). Intermediate categories such as 'minimal improvement' and 'marked improvement' were not used because they were regarded as difficult to evaluate. Less than one in fifty couples who applied for therapy were turned down and this was on the basis of three criteria: 1) psychosis in one partner; 2) a partner with a vested interest in remaining sexually dysfunctional or maintaining his or her partner's dysfunction; and 3) medical conditions that minimised or precluded the possibility that sex therapy would be successful. The follow-up study of 226 patients relied on a standard set of mainly open-ended questions (not provided by Kolodny). Kolodny (1981) agreed that Masters and Johnson's follow-up phone calls to patients were often a form of therapy. He estimated that the calls lasted an average of twenty minutes and that 85% of their patients received 'no more than four phone calls a year' (Kolodny 1981, 310).

In sum, Kolodny's (1981) article did provide much of the information that Zilbergeld and Evans (1980) sought about Masters and Johnson's (1970) work. However, the very fact that Kolodny's reply was necessary is significant. Its substance indicates that many of Zilbergeld and Evans' concerns about the inadequacy of Masters and Johnson's methodology and reporting were basically justified. Furthermore, it took some eleven years after *Human Sexual Inadequacy* was first published for this methodological information to be made publicly available. This casts doubt on Masters and Johnson's (1970, 351) claim that replication could be used to assess the reported successes of their treatment program. Without the sort of information provided by Kolodny (1981), attempts at replication would have been vitiated and Masters and Johnson's (1970) claims of therapeutic success could not have been independently assessed. Without the possibility of independent assessment, Masters and Johnson's claims basically rested on their scientific and clinical authority. This was apparently enough for many people to accept their claims.

Kolodny (1981) also failed to answer one of Zilbergeld and Evans' (1980) most important criticisms of Masters and Johnson (1970). He did not provide any information on the criteria which Masters and Johnson used to determine failure and nonfailure for the specific sexual dysfunctions they treated. After reviewing Kolodny's (1981) article, Evans and Zilbergeld (1983, 304) lamented that 'Until the Masters and Johnson Institute provides comparable criteria [to other researchers] their work cannot be properly evaluated or replicated, despite their own emphasis on the need for such replication.'

When Masters and Johnson remained silent about their outcome criteria, Zilbergeld publicly attacked them in a series of lectures. He particularly focused on the lack of a criterion for the nonfailure of treatment for female orgasmic dysfunction. He wondered whether nonfailure meant that a woman could now have an orgasm 100%, 50%, 10%, or some other percentage of the times she had sex. After Zilbergeld attacked Masters and Johnson on this issue at the annual meeting of the Society for the Scientific Study of Sex in 1982, Zilbergeld, Masters, and a number of associates met to discuss the criteria of failure and nonfailure. Zilbergeld took notes of what Masters said, read them back to him for confirmation and Masters agreed they were accurate (Heidenry 1997, 285). Masters reportedly said that 'therapeutic success was predicated upon a non-orgasmic woman having one orgasm during the two weeks of therapy and one orgasm during the next five years' (Irvine 1990a, 200). This criterion seemed to explain Masters and Johnson's incredible treatment results: two orgasms in over five years was regarded as a cure.

Masters later denied this was his criterion but a number of other people at the meeting confirmed what he had said. He again refused to discuss the matter until he could do so in a scientific setting (Irvine 1990a, 200; Heidenry 1997, 285). In the meantime, Dr Sallie Schumacher, who trained with Masters and Johnson and collaborated on *Human Sexual Inadequacy*, revealed that as 'far as she understood there were no clear outcome criteria' (Heidenry 1997, 286). If this was true, it meant that the sole means of determining failure and nonfailure was the clinical judgement of the researchers themselves and this may well have been biased (Schover and Leiblum 1994, 18). Zilbergeld speculated that 'Masters and Johnson had concealed their outcome statistics in order to legitimate their controversial work. Unless they reported excellent results... their whole endeavour would have been open to challenge' (Irvine 1990a, 201).

In 1983, at the sixth World Congress of Sexology in Washington, Masters finally released outcome criteria that he claimed he and Johnson had used for each type of dysfunction (Brody 1983; Wolinsky 1983; Bancroft 1989, 493). It was issued only after a series of very public attacks which threatened their scientific reputations, the credibility of their work and the marketability of their sex therapy. It also came some thirteen years after *Human Sexual Inadequacy* was first published, and led to their admission that their work was not 'without significant flaws' (Wolinsky 1983, 2). The researchers, who accepted that replication was the 'impeccable clinical yardstick' which could 'be applied without reservation' to their own work, had effectively protected that work from replication by withholding essential information about it for as long as possible. And when they did release the criterion of treatment nonfailure for female orgasmic dysfunction, it was probably not surprising that it turned out to be much more stringent than the original criterion that Masters reportedly gave Zilbergeld. The latest criterion was that a woman had to be orgasmic in at least 50% of her sexual opportunities to be classified as a nonfailure (Brody 1983; Wolinsky 1983; Heidenry 1997, 287).

Despite many valid criticisms of Masters and Johnson, however, their sex therapy was nevertheless credited with helping many couples with 'sexual dysfunctions' to improve their sex lives (Bancroft 1989, 461; Irvine 1990a, 199). Their therapy seemed particularly well suited to helping people without major psychiatric or medical illnesses, and whose main problems stemmed from sexual ignorance, inexperience, anxiety or negative attitudes about sex (Masters and Johnson 1970, 21; LoPiccolo 1994, 5; Maurice 2001). Their reported low treatment failure rates were also likely to have been, in part, a reflection of their non-representative patient sample. Masters and Johnson (1970, 356–7) primarily worked with highly educated 'middle class' couples (many of whom were health professionals) who were highly motivated to try and reverse their sexual symptomatology (sexual dysfunctions). Masters and Johnson (1970, 358) themselves stated that:

> With the multiple facets of involuntary selectivity in the clinical research population running entirely in support of the treatment program, failure rates should always be evaluated with the conscious realization that Foundation personnel have had every possible advantage in treatment opportunity during the last 11 years.

Masters and Johnson's (1970) therapy regime, however, was not a panacea for sexual problems, and their hope that sexual inadequacy would become obsolete within a decade was far too optimistic. Results of controlled outcome studies of sex therapy's effectiveness were more sobering than the original results claimed by Masters and Johnson (1970). According to Bancroft (1989, 462):

> It has become clear, even to those working in the USA, that the extreme optimism of the early 1970s was deceptive. A more realistic and less simplistic view is beginning to emerge which recognises the considerable heterogeneity of problems that present for sex therapy, with their widely differing therapeutic needs and prognoses.

This conclusion has been reaffirmed by more recent reviews of outcome research on sex therapy (see, for example, Hawton 1991; LoPiccolo 1994; Schover and Leiblum 1994; Donahey and Miller 2000, 221). There is also something of a consensus among sex therapists that 'all the easy cases have gone' and that Masters and Johnson's (1970) therapeutic approach is inadequate for treating 'today's typical sex therapy patients' (LoPiccolo 1994, 5; Schover and Leiblum 1994, 18; Wiederman 1998). Many of these patients present with such problems as 'major psychopathology, substance abuse, histories of abuse as a child or spouse, and extreme relationship conflict' (Schover and Leiblum 1994, 18–19). Brief, behaviourally oriented sex therapy usually has poor treatment outcomes with these groups of patients (Schover and Leiblum 1994, 19).

SEX THERAPY AS AN INSTITUTION OF SOCIAL CONTROL

Finally, Masters and Johnson's (1970) sex therapy program can be criticised for attempting to 'normalise' patients' sexual functioning in line with its own socially constructed standards of sexual health and response. Masters and Johnson believed that healthy sexual functioning is functioning which conforms to their 'universal' model of the human sexual response cycle and which enables the 'satisfactory' performance of penile-vaginal intercourse. They regarded this standard as a 'natural' norm which they had scientifically discovered in the course of their objective and value free research. In previous chapters, however, I pointed out that Masters and Johnson had failed to show that this standard was natural, universal or objective. It was argued that Masters and Johnson presupposed rather than discovered this standard and that it is based on strongly essentialist and hetero-coital assumptions about sexuality. Masters and Johnson nevertheless took this as their norm of healthy sexual functioning and defined sexual dysfunctions as pathological deviations from the norm. Defining conditions as health or medical problems, however, involves making value judgements. If the standard of normal sexual functioning is a social construction based on dominant cultural values, then sex therapy can be regarded as an institution of social control. This is because it identifies, labels and treats aspects of human sexuality as dysfunctional in order to promote conformity to this standard.

Drawing on the work of Conrad and Schneider (1985, ch.9), I have argued that this has a number of important consequences (Morrow 1994, 32). Firstly, sexologists, such as Masters and Johnson, tend to medicalise and mystify the meaning of people's experiences so that people with otherwise satisfying sex lives might come to regard themselves or their partners as having sexual problems if they do not have rigid erections, penetrable vaginas, 'mature' ejaculations or coital orgasms. Yet Masters and Johnson seem to make little effort in explaining to people that many of these 'problems' — which are defined in relation to the 'satisfactory' performance of heterosexual coitus — might disappear without the 'coital imperative', and if coitus ceased to be the sole or primary measure of sexual health. For Masters and Johnson (1970), however, 'satisfactory' penile-vaginal intercourse is the unquestioned goal of their therapy program (Everaerd 2001, 13967). When other forms of stimulation, such as manual stimulation, are taught to patients they are done less as ends in themselves and more as 'bridges' to accomplishing 'satisfactory' penis in vagina sex (Reiss 1990, 171).

Secondly, the medicalisation of 'deviant' sexual response contributes to the individualisation of sexual problems. The cause of the problem is believed to lie within the individual (or for Masters and Johnson 'the couple'). This means it is the individual (or couple) who needs to be 'cured' and changed rather than examining the way in which power relations and inequalities within society might impact on people's sexual experiences and relationships (Blanc 2001). In an interesting Australian study, Berg (1986, 170), for example, pointed out how 'women's economic, social and emotional dependency' on men militated against women's sexual equality in relationships in terms of their ability to consistently reach orgasm. Irvine (1990a, 199) has made a similar point. She argues that Masters and Johnson's (1970) version of sex therapy will never be more than a 'band-aid solution' for sexual problems. This is because it does not 'touch the source of the most intractable sexual problems of heterosexuals: fear, anger, boredom, overwork and lack of time, inequality in the relationship, prior sexual assault on the woman, and differential socialization and sexual scripts' (Irvine 1990a, 199).

Thirdly, the individualisation and medicalisation of sexual 'problems' makes their management compatible with commodification, in the form of private fee-for-service sex therapy (Morrow 1994, 32). As Irvine (1990a, 199) puts it, 'In sex therapy, the "cure" is orgasm, not social change. And this is vital because orgasms can be marketed in a profit-making system, while social change cannot.' Not only is sex therapy's emphasis much more on the 'cure' rather than prevention of sexual problems but high fees and associated costs restrict access to therapy for many people. In 1970, for example, Masters and Johnson charged patients $2,500 for a fortnight of treatment and five year follow-up. Patients also had to absorb accommodation and travel costs and loss of earnings during that time (Bejin 1986a, 185). By 1989, the average fee had increased to $6,000 (Irvine 1990a, 318). Masters and Johnson did provide free care to patients from 1959 to 1964 but from 1965 they introduced an adjusted fee schedule: 50% of their patients paid the full fee ($2,500); 25% of their patients paid an adjusted fee ($1,250); and 25% of patients received free care (Masters and Johnson 1970, 356; Lehrman 1976, 90). Belliveau and Richter (1971, 85) point out, however, that 'Even with an adjusted fee schedule, patients have tended to be middle class or above.'

Bejin (1986a, 185) has also questioned Masters and Johnson's apparently altruistic motives in the provision of free treatment. He says:

> These 'good deeds' are less 'gratuitous' than they appear. They provide therapists with three interesting possibilities: 1) to try out new modes of treatment; 2) to see unusual and hence scientifically 'interesting' cases; 3) to anticipate the preparation of therapeutic methods applicable to future 'markets' with a less well-to-do and less educated clientele, who one day ought to benefit from the 'democritization' (sic) of these treatments. (Bejin 1986a, 185)

Finally, medicalising and individualising sexual 'problems' depoliticises them. Szasz (1981, xii) points out, for example, that moral and political aspects of sexuality become masked by medical labels. In particular, there has been a substantial failure to challenge Masters and Johnson's norms of sexual health and thus a failure to help many people recognise and consider alternative viewpoints and sexual practices. Masters and Johnson's clinical norms have been generally upheld while thousands of individuals came to believe they were sexually dysfunctional and sought out sex therapy for their 'problems.' In terms of C. Wright Mills's (1970) famous formulation, a 'public issue' affecting vast numbers of people has been turned into the 'personal troubles' of individuals.

CONCLUSION

This chapter provided a critique of the nature and effectiveness of Masters and Johnson's (1970) sex therapy program. The chapter argued that, rather than being highly original, Masters and Johnson's sex therapy program was largely based on the unacknowledged principles and techniques of behaviour therapy. Their therapeutic approach was different from earlier approaches, however, in that it mainly involved treatment of a couple by male and female co-therapists (such as a doctor and psychologist); brief, intensive therapy; and the integration of specific sexual dysfunction treatment strategies into an overall treatment package.

The chapter pointed out that Masters and Johnson aimed to treat marital relationships as their patients, and that the immediate goal of their therapy program was to return sex to its 'natural context'. This latter term was not defined but, to the extent that it ignored the social and psychological aspects of sexual functioning, it seems to be a misconceived and unattainable goal. In practice, however, it meant enabling couples to 'satisfactorily' perform heterosexual intercourse. Masters and Johnson believed that sexual dysfunctions were largely caused by ignorance of sexual physiology and sociocultural deprivation, and they discriminated between current and historical causes of sexual dysfunction. However, they generally focused on the personal troubles of their patients, and largely neglected to analyse the social and political context within which individuals sexually functioned and related to others. Their therapy program itself was mainly concerned with providing couples with sex education, advice, and permission to enjoy sexual activity, as well as teaching specific behavioural techniques for treating particular types of dysfunction.

In their book, *Human Sexual Inadequacy*, Masters and Johnson (1970) reported on their 'new' short-term, intensive way of treating sexual dysfunctions. They claimed their treatment was highly effective and had an overall failure rate of only 20%. I argued that their work received an enthusiastic and largely uncritical reception. Their work contributed to the development of sex therapy as a new 'profession', the proliferation of thousands of sex clinics across the United States, and expectations that sexual dysfunctions could be 'substantially eliminated' within the next decade.

Drawing primarily on Zilbergeld and Evans's (1980) work, I then argued that Masters and Johnson's (1970) study of their sex therapy's effectiveness (the largest such study ever reported) was so full of methodological problems and poor reporting that it is impossible to know how effective their therapy was. Despite the doubts, however, their therapy program was still credited with 'successfully' treating many people with 'sexual dysfunctions'. Their therapy seemed to be most 'successful' with patients whose sexual 'problems' were due to ignorance, inexperience, anxiety, and negative attitudes toward sex. It was not a panacea for sexual dysfunctions, though, and it appears to have become less 'successful' in treating contemporary sex therapy patients.

The chapter concluded by focusing on the unacknowledged way that Masters and Johnson's sex therapy program operated as an institution of social control. Its operations served to 'normalise' patients' sexual responses in line with socially constructed standards of health and normality. I argued that, in doing so, the program medicalised, individualised and depoliticised individuals' sexual 'problems' while responding to them with commodified treatments and 'cures'.

8   Conclusion

The primary aim of this book was to provide a sociological analysis and critique of the conceptual foundations and practice of Masters and Johnson's (1966; 1970) sex research and therapy. This was accomplished primarily through an internal critique of the main themes and ideas in *Human Sexual Response* and *Human Sexual Inadequacy*. There has previously been no overall, systematic, book-length sociological account of these works and their interrelationship. The existing sociological literature about them is small, fragmented and selective in its focus. In addition, the research findings from this literature have often been non-cumulative. The lack of previous sociological attention to Masters and Johnson cannot be explained by arguing that the sociology of sex first developed late in the postwar era and was too immature to provide critical analyses of their work. No comprehensive history of the sociology of sex appears to exist. However, the sociology of sex has a long history, and I documented much of this from the 1840s to 1960, focusing particularly on U.S. sociology. This history is largely unknown by sociologists mainly because the rise of the classical canon in sociology altered many sociologists' conceptions of their discipline, their discipline's history, and the kind of topics that were thought worthy of study. The lack of sociological attention to Masters and Johnson's sex research and therapy was mainly due to the influence of the classical canon, the way in which their work was defined in hegemonic biomedical and clinical terms, and the perceived high quality and importance of their work.

I outlined and criticised the dominant essentialist theoretical perspective on human sexuality which Masters and Johnson worked with. I argued for the use of a modified form of social constructionism as a viable perspective for guiding the critical analysis of Masters and Johnson's scientific and clinical work. Social constructionism is a useful perspective for challenging positivist and common sense accounts of science and for thinking about taken for granted issues in new ways. However, it needs to be grounded in explicitly realist philosophical assumptions if it is to avoid the serious problems that are otherwise generated by the view that reality is unknowable and that truth is relative to social context.

After evaluating the major theoretical perspectives on human sexuality, I turned to Masters and Johnson's laboratory research. Contrary to popular belief, Masters and Johnson were not the first researchers to directly study human sexual response. However, they aimed to collect definitive scientific information about it which would demonstrate the objectivity and usefulness of sex research, and provide a baseline of what was normal for understanding and treating human sexual inadequacy. Masters and Johnson's approach was modelled on that of scientific medicine and they framed their research to address pressing public concerns about divorce and family break down in U.S. society. This helped to provide legitimacy for their project, and further their research and clinical objectives.

After some important initial research with prostitutes, Masters and Johnson recruited 694 people for their laboratory research on human sexual response. This selective sample was unrepresentative of U.S. society. It was chosen mainly for its convenience and because the research participants were most likely to sexually respond in the ways that Masters and Johnson required. After eleven years of their laboratory work, Masters and Johnson published an account of this research in their famous book *Human Sexual Response*. Their main research finding was that male and female sexual response are so similar that they can be understood as occurring within a single four stage human sexual response cycle. The publication of their book was a major commercial and cultural event with profound and wide ranging impacts. Their research findings were generally accepted as scientific fact by most audiences, although some critics were concerned about the methods of their research.

Masters and Johnson's (1966) model of the human sexual response cycle, however, was far more problematic than most people realised. It was not a wholly objective account of their research findings at all. Masters and Johnson were under pressure to produce new and original findings on human sexual response to help justify their laboratory research. This may have led them to falsely claim that they were the first to develop a four stage model of human sexual response. Yet, such a model had already been developed by Albert Moll (1912), and Masters and Johnson were aware of his work. Masters and Johnson also adhered to a problematic essentialist perspective on sexuality which led them to assume the existence of a biological sex drive, to ignore the issue of sexual desire in their model, and to interpret sexual physiology as if heterosexual copulation was the only 'biologically correct' way to respond to sexual excitement. There was also a range of inconsistencies between their own data on sexual response and their model of the human sexual response cycle. Some of these inconsistencies appear to be explicable in terms of their ideological emphasis on the sexual similarities of males and females, the way they tried to force specific findings into their model of sexual response, and their arguments with the Freudians over the anatomical distinctness of clitoral and vaginal orgasms in women. Masters and Johnson emphasised the sexual similarities of males and females in their research even though they 'found' both similarities and differences. Their emphasis on sexual similarity appears to be ideological and connected to their belief that a recognition of sexual similarity would provide a basis for equal and harmonious sexual relationships between men and women. Masters and Johnson also claimed that two of the key differences between males and females are that only females are capable of multiple orgasm, and that only males are capable of ejaculation. Yet, Masters and Johnson did not investigate the topic of male multiple orgasm, found no evidence of it in their sample of men, and wrongly concluded that it did not exist in the human male. They also conflated orgasm and ejaculation in men despite earlier research by Kinsey and colleagues (1948) pointing out the differences between these physiological processes. In addition, Masters and Johnson dismissed reports of female ejaculation among some of their research participants because they were convinced it could not happen and that the women were misinterpreting their own experiences. It is now known that some women, at least, do expel fluid (which is not urine) from their urethras during orgasm.

Despite the various problems with Masters and Johnson's model of the human sexual response cycle, it was nevertheless used in their sex therapy program, along with the ability to 'satisfactorily' perform heterosexual coitus, as norms of healthy sexual functioning. Deviations from these norms would constitute sexual dysfunctions, and Masters and Johnson produced a new and influential way of classifying them.

However, their model of the human sexual response cycle has limited generalisabilty in providing a set of clinical norms (of healthy sexual functioning) for the general population. This is because Masters and Johnson conducted their laboratory research in such a way that it would confirm their pre-existing ideas about human sexual response. They also generally ignored the way that differences between their unrepresentative research sample and the wider U.S. population might be relevant to understanding human sexual functioning. Moreover, their nosology of sexual dysfunction had a strong hetero-coital bias (connected to their strongly essentialist assumptions about human sexuality), it unnecessarily pathologised deviant sexual response, it contained unexplained or unjustified gender biases in the classification of sexual dysfunction, it assumed that sexual dysfunctions are intrinsically sexual problems, and it had no way of coping with sexual problems that did not involve sexual dysfunction. Notwithstanding the various problems with this nosology, it was nevertheless incorporated into their sex therapy program and became very influential within sexology.

Masters and Johnson's (1970) sex therapy program was thought to be highly original but was largely based on the unacknowledged principles and techniques of behaviour therapy. It differed from earlier therapeutic approaches, however, in that it involved treatment of a couple by a couple, brief intensive therapy, and specific treatment regimes for each of the sexual dysfunctions. Masters and Johnson treated marital relationships as their patients and believed that sexual dysfunctions were largely caused by ignorance of sexual physiology and sociocultural deprivation. However, they were more concerned with the personal troubles of their patients without analysing the wider social and political context of their patients' lives. Their therapy program aimed to return sex to its 'natural context' (an undefined state) which effectively meant assisting couples to have 'satisfactory' heterosexual intercourse.

Masters and Johnson's (1970) book *Human Sexual Inadequacy* reported on their 'new' approach to sex therapy. In the largest ever outcome study of treatment for sexual dysfunction, involving 790 patients and five year patient follow-up data, Masters and Johnson claimed an overall failure rate of only 20%. Their work was hailed as 'revolutionary' and 'epoch-making'. People rushed to train as sex therapists with Masters and Johnson, existing therapists began incorporating Masters and Johnson's methods into their own therapeutic repertoires, and sex therapy clinics began proliferating across the United States. Expectations were heightened that sex therapy might virtually eliminate sexual dysfunctions in the population. The lack of critical scrutiny of Masters and Johnson's work was probably due to their reputations as rigorous scientists, the inaccessibility of their writing style, their self-critical presentation, the dependency of other sexologists on their 'pioneering' work, and lower standards in sexology (compared with more established disciplines) for the publication and presentation of research findings.

When Masters and Johnson's claims about their sex therapy's effectiveness were closely examined, serious problems began to emerge. Major methodological problems with their study and the poor reporting of information meant that it was impossible to know how effective their therapy was, and their study could not be replicated. Masters and Johnson's therapy program was nevertheless credited with 'successfully' treating many people with 'sexual dysfunctions'. However, it seemed to be most 'successful' with those who were sexually anxious and inexperienced. It did not prove to be a panacea for sexual dysfunction and it appears to be less 'successful' in treating contemporary sex therapy patients.

Masters and Johnson's sex therapy program was also concerned with normalising patients' sexual responses to socially constructed standards of healthy sexual functioning. It apparently did not encourage patients to question these norms, or to consider alternative sexual possibilities and practices. In this respect, it operated as an institution of social control which reinforced dominant essentialist and hetero-coital views of sexuality. Culturally disapproved sexual responses were medicalised and individualised, the social context of sexual problems was often neglected (particularly issues concerning power and social inequality), and individualised treatments and 'cures' were marketed and sold as commodities. This worked to the economic benefit of the therapists, and even the free provision of treatment had unacknowledged benefits for them.

Finally, the critique of Masters and Johnson's work has a number of implications for contemporary sex therapy. Firstly, it is important that sex therapists do not uncritically use Masters and Johnson's (1966) model of the human sexual response cycle as a universal norm of healthy sexual functioning which everyone, in all circumstances, is expected to approximate. Deviations in sexual response from this model are not necessarily pathological, and individuals may desire and value, or, at least, not be concerned about sexual responses that do not conform to this model. Similarly, sex therapists need to avoid regarding 'satisfactory' hetero-coital sex as the natural and unquestioned norm of healthy sexual functioning. This has not been demonstrated and it normatively privileges hetero-coital sex over other forms of sexual expression.

Secondly, Masters and Johnson's (1970) nosology of sexual dysfunction is so arbitrary, selective, inconsistent and confusing that it should be fundamentally re-constructed. Sex therapists need to be more aware that sexual problems can come in a wide variety of forms and are not reducible to sexual dysfunctions; that sexual responses which deviate from social expectations are not necessarily sexual dysfunctions; that patients may not regard sexual dysfunctions as sexual problems; and that apparently technical diagnostic terms may stigmatise and cause distress to those who are labelled with them.

Thirdly, sex therapy needs to look beyond the personal troubles of patients, and try to examine how these troubles might be part of wider public issues which arise from the structure and culture of their society. This would not only enrich therapists' understandings of sexual problems, it might also lead to interventions that go beyond the individual (or couple) level, and lead to greater emphasis on the prevention of such problems. (However, in order to avoid possible problems with professional dominance and social control, more democratic and participatory forms of interaction may be required than the more traditional hierarchical relationships between professionals and clients).

Fourthly, sex therapists need to be more reflexive and sociologically aware if they are to avoid acting as agents of social control. If therapists are to empower their patients to understand and better deal with their sexual problems, then they will need to help patients question socially constructed standards of healthy and unhealthy sexual functioning, and to consider a wider range of sexual choices than might be normatively accepted within their society.

Fifthly, sex therapy needs much better treatment outcome studies than Masters and Johnson provided. This requires much more careful attention to methodological and reporting issues. Good quality outcome studies are vital if sex therapists are to have confidence in their methods and provide the most efficacious forms of treatment.

Finally, when sex therapy can be effective, sex therapists need to consider whether their therapy is best delivered as a commodity or as a non-commodified service. While Masters and Johnson did provide some free and cut-price treatment to patients, their therapy, on the whole, was an expensive commodity beyond the financial reach of many people. If sex therapy can truly make a difference to people's lives, then issues of access and economic inequality will also have to be addressed.

References

Abercrombie, N., Hill, S., and Turner, B. S. (1994). *The Penguin Dictionary of Sociology*, 3rd edn, London: Penguin.
—— (2000). *The Penguin Dictionary of Sociology*, 4th edn, London: Penguin.
Abramson, P. and Pinkerton, S. D. (1995). *With Pleasure: Thoughts on the nature of human sexuality*, New York: Oxford University Press.
American Psychiatric Association (1980). *Diagnostic and Statistical Manual of Mental Disorders*, 3rd edn, Washington, DC: American Psychiatric Association.
—— (1987). *Diagnostic and Statistical Manual of Mental Disorders*, 3rd edn, rev., Washington, DC: American Psychiatric Association.
—— (1994). *Diagnostic and Statistical Manual of Mental Disorders*, 4th edn, Washington, DC: American Psychiatric Association.
—— (2000). *Diagnostic and Statistical Manual of Mental Disorders*, 4th edn, Text Revision, Washington, DC: American Psychiatric Association.
Archer, M. (1998). 'Introduction: realism in the social sciences' in Archer, M., Bhaskar, R., Collier, A., Lawson, T. and Norrie, A. (eds.) *Critical Realism: Essential readings*, London: Routledge.
Assiter, A. (1996). *Enlightened Women: Modernist feminism in a postmodern age*, London: Routledge.
Azevedo, J. (1997). *Mapping Reality: An Evolutionary realist methodology for the natural and social sciences*, Albany: State University of New York Press.
Baert, P. (1998). *Social Theory in the Twentieth Century*, Cambridge: Polity Press.
Bancroft, J. (1986). 'Sex therapy' in Bloch, S. (ed.) *An Introduction to the Psychotherapies*, 2nd edn, Oxford: Oxford University Press.
—— (1989). *Human Sexuality and Its Problems*, 2nd edn, Edinburgh: Churchill Livingstone.
Bannister, R. C. (1987). *Sociology and Scientism: The American quest for objectivity, 1880–1940*, Chapel Hill: University of North Carolina Press.
Beach, F. A. (1956) 'Characteristics of masculine "sex drive"' in Jones, M. R. (ed.) *Nebraska Symposium on Motivation*, Lincoln: University of Nebraska Press.
Beaton Peterson, G. and Peterson, L. R. (1973). 'Sexism in the treatment of sexual dysfunction', *The Family Coordinator*, 22, 4, 397–404.
Bejin, A. (1986a). 'The decline of the psycho-analyst and the rise of the sexologist' in Aries, P. and Bejin, A. (eds.) *Western Sexuality*, Oxford: Basil Blackwell.
—— (1986b). 'The influence of the sexologists and sexual democracy' in Aries, P. and Bejin, A. (eds.) *Western Sexuality*, Oxford: Basil Blackwell.

Belliveau, F. and Richter, L. (1971). *Understanding Human Sexual Inadequacy*, London: Hodder & Stoughton.

Berg, R. (1986). 'Sexuality: why do women come off second best?' in Grieve, N. and Burns, A. (eds.) *Australian Women: New feminist perspectives*, Melbourne: Oxford University Press.

Berger, P. L. and Luckmann, T. (1966). *The Social Construction of Reality*, Garden City, New York: Doubleday.

Berliner, H. S. (1984). 'Scientific medicine since Flexner' in Salmon, J. W. (ed.) *Alternative Medicines: Popular and policy perspectives*, New York: Tavistock.

Blackburn, S. (1996). *Oxford Dictionary of Philosophy*, Oxford: Oxford University Press.

Blanc, A. K. (2001). 'The effect of power in sexual relationships on sexual and reproductive health: an examination of the evidence', *Studies in Family Planning*, 32, 3, 189–213.

Blau, P. M. (ed.) (1966). *Cumulative Index to the American Journal of Sociology, Volumes 1–70, 1895–1965*, Chicago: University of Chicago Press.

Bottomore, T. (1984). *Sociology and Socialism*, Brighton: Wheatsheaf.

Bowman, C. C. (1949). 'Cultural ideology and heterosexual reality: a preface to sociological research', *American Sociological Review*, 14, 624–33.

Boyle, M. (1993). 'Sexual dysfunction or heterosexual dysfunction?', *Feminism and Psychology*, 3, 1, 73–88.

—— (1994). 'Gender, science and sexual dysfunction' in Sarbin, T. R. and Kitsuse, J. I. (eds.) *Constructing the Social*, London: Sage.

Brecher, E. M. (1970). *The Sex Researchers*, London: Andre Deutsch.

Brecher, R. and Brecher, E. (eds.) (1967). *An Analysis of Human Sexual Response*, London: Andre Deutsch.

—— (eds.) (1968). *An Analysis of Human Sexual Response*, London: Panther.

Brickell, C. (2006) 'The sociological construction of gender and sexuality', *Sociological Review*, 54, 1, 87–113.

Brody, J. E. (1983). 'Masters and Johnson defend pioneer sex therapy research', *New York Times*, 27 May.

Bromberg, W. (1943). 'The effects of the war on crime', *American Sociological Review*, 8, 6, 685–91.

Bromley, D. D. and Britten, F. H. (1938). *Youth and Sex: A study of 1300 college Students*, New York: Harper & Bros.

Bullough, V. L. (1985). 'Problems of research on a delicate topic: a personal view', *The Journal of Sex Research*, 21, 4, 375–86.

—— (1994a). *Science in the Bedroom: A history of sex research*, New York: Basic Books.

—— (1994b). 'The development of sexology in the USA in the early twentieth century' in Porter, R. and Teich, M. (eds.) *Sexual Knowledge, Sexual Science: The history of attitudes to sexuality*, Cambridge: Cambridge University Press.

—— (1994c). 'Freud, Sigmund' in Bullough, V. L. and Bullough, B. (eds.) *Human Sexuality: An encyclopedia*, New York: Garland Publishing.

—— (1994d). 'Masters, William Howell' in Bullough, V. L. and Bullough, B. (eds.) *Human Sexuality: An encyclopedia*, New York: Garland Publishing.

Burgess, E. W. (1926). 'The romantic impulse and family disorganization', *Survey*, 57, 290–4.

—— (1939a). 'Three pioneers in the study of sex', *Marriage and Family Living* 1, pages 76 and 95.

—— (1939b). 'The influence of Sigmund Freud upon sociology in the United States', *American Journal of Sociology*, 45, 3, 356–74.

——— (1942). 'The effect of war on the American family', *American Journal of Sociology*, 48, 3, 343–52.

Burgess, E. W. and Cottrell, Jr., L. S. (1939). *Predicting Success or Failure in Marriage*, New York: Prentice-Hall.

Burgess, E. W. and Wallin, P. (1953). *Engagement and Marriage*, Chicago: J.B. Lippincott Co.

Cadden, V. (1978). 'The psychiatrists versus Masters and Johnson' in LoPiccolo, J. and LoPiccolo, L. (eds.) *Handbook of Sex Therapy*, New York: Plenum Press.

Calderone, M. S. (1983). 'Theoretical issues in sexology: education for sexuality' in Davis, C.M. (ed.) *Challenges in Sexual Science*, Iowa: Society for the Scientific Study of Sex.

Capra, F. (1983). *The Turning Point: Science, Society and the rising culture*, London: Flamingo.

Cohn-Bendit, D., Duteuil, J-P., Gerard, B. and Granautier, B. (1969). 'Why sociologists?' in Cockburn, A. and Blackburn, R. (eds.) *Student Power: Problems, diagnosis, action,* Harmondsworth: Penguin.

Collison, P. and Webber, S. (1971). 'British sociology 1950–1970: a journal analysis', *Sociological Review*, 19, 521–42.

Comte, A. (1975 [1851–1854]). *Auguste Comte and Positivism: The essential writings*, Lenzer, G. (ed.), Chicago: University of Chicago Press.

Connell, R. W. (1997). 'Why is classical theory classical?', *American Journal of Sociology* 102, 6, 1511–57.

Connell, R. W. and Dowsett, G. W. (1992). '"The unclean motion of the generative parts": frameworks in Western thought on sexuality' in Connell, R. W. and Dowsett, G. W. (eds.) *Rethinking Sex: Social theory and sexuality research*, Melbourne: Melbourne University Press.

Conrad, P. (1992). 'Medicalization and social control', *Annual Review of Sociology*, 18, 209–32.

——— (2005). 'The shifting engines of medicalization', *Journal of Health and Social Behavior*, 46, 1, 3–14.

Conrad, P. and Schneider, J. W. (1985). *Deviance and Medicalization: From badness to sickness*, Columbus: Merrill.

Craib, I. (1997). 'Social constructionism as a social psychosis', *Sociology*, 31, 1, 1–15.

Cressey, P. G. (1969 [1932]). *The Taxi-Dance Hall*, Montclair, New Jersey: Patterson Smith.

Danermark, B. (2001). 'Interdisciplinary research and critical realism - the example of disability research', Swedish Institute for Disability Research, Orebro University.

Darling, C. A., Davidson, Sr., J. K., and Conway-Welch, C. (1990). 'Female ejaculation: Perceived origins, the Grafenberg spot/area, and sexual responsiveness', *Archives of Sexual Behavior*, 19, 1, 29–47.

Davenport, W. (1968). 'Sexual patterns in a south-west Pacific society' in Brecher, R. and Brecher, E. (eds.) *An Analysis of Human Sexual Response*, London: Panther.

Davis, C. M. (ed.) (1983). *Challenges in Sexual Science*, Iowa: Society for the Scientific Study of Sex.

Davis, D. and Whitten, R. G. (1987). 'The cross-cultural study of human sexuality', *Annual Review of Anthropology*, 16, 69–98.

Davis, K. (1936). 'Jealousy and sexual property', *Social Forces*, 14, 395–405.

——— (1937). 'The sociology of prostitution', *American Sociological Review*, 2, 744–55.

—— (1939a). 'Illegitimacy and the social structure', *American Journal of Sociology*, 45, 215–33.

—— (1939b). 'The forms of illegitimacy', *Social Forces*, 18, 77–89.

—— (1959). 'The myth of functional analysis as a special method in sociology and anthropology', *American Sociological Review*, 24, 6, 757–72.

—— (1976). 'Sexual behavior' in Merton, R. K. and Nisbet, R. (eds.) *Contemporary Social Problems*, 4th edn, New York: Harcourt Brace Jovanovich.

Davis, K. B. (1929). *Factors in the Sex Life of Twenty-Two Hundred Women*, New York: Harper & Bros.

Davison, G. C. and Neale, J. M. (1994). *Abnormal Psychology*, 6th edn, New York: John Wiley & Sons.

Dead or Alive? (2001). Site updated on 18 February 2001, viewed on 23 March 2001, <http://www.dead-or-alive.org/dead.nsf/mnames-nf/Masters+William>.

Degler, C. N. (1984). 'What ought to be and what was: women's sexuality in the nineteenth century' in Leavitt, J. W. (ed.) *Women and Health in America*, Madison: University of Wisconsin Press.

Dein, S. (1993/1994). 'Culture and sexuality', *British Medical Anthropology Review*, 22, 22–30.

DeLamater, J. (1981). 'The social control of sexuality', *Annual Review of Sociology*, 7, 263–90.

DeLamater, J. D. and Hyde, J. S. (1998). 'Essentialism vs. social constructionism in the study of human sexuality', *The Journal of Sex Research*, 35, 1, 10–18.

DeLora, J. S. and Warren, C. A. B. (1977). *Understanding Sexual Interaction*, Boston: Houghton Mifflin.

de Visser, R. O., Smith, A. M. A., Rissel, C. E., Richters, J. and Grulich, A. E. (2003). 'Sex in Australia: heterosexual experience and recent heterosexual encounters among a representative sample of adults', *Australian and New Zealand Journal of Public Health*, 27, 2, 146–54.

Devitt, M. (1991). *Realism and Truth*, 2nd edn, Oxford: Blackwell.

Dickinson, R. L. and Beam, L. (1970 [1931]). *A Thousand Marriages*, Westport, Connecticut: Greenwood Press.

Donahey, K. M. and Miller, S. D. (2000). 'Applying a common factors perspective to sex therapy', *Journal of Sex Education and Therapy*, 25, 4, 221–30.

Dunn, M. E. and Trost, J. E. (1989). 'Male multiple orgasms: a descriptive study', *Archives of Sexual Behavior*, 18, 5, 377–87.

Durkheim, E. (1963 [1897]). *Incest: The nature and origin of the taboo*, trans. by Sagarin, E., New York: Lyle Stuart.

—— (1964 [1894]). *The Rules of Sociological Method*, 8th edn, trans. by Solovay, S. A. and Mueller, J. H., New York: Free Press.

—— (1970 [1897]). *Suicide: A study in sociology*, trans. by Spaulding, J. A. and Simpson, G., London: Routledge & Kegan Paul.

—— (1976 [1912]). *The Elementary Forms of the Religious Life*, 2nd edn, trans. by Swain, J. W., London: George Allen & Unwin.

—— (1979 [1911]). 'A discussion on sex education' in Pickering, W. S. F. (ed.) *Durkheim: Essays on morals and education*, London: Routledge & Kegan Paul.

Ehrenreich, B., Hess, E., and Jacobs, G. (1987). *Re-Making Love: The feminization of sex*, New York: Anchor.

Ehrmann, W. (1959). *Premarital Dating Behavior*, New York: Holt.

—— (1963). 'Social determinants of human sexual behavior' in Winokur, G. (ed.) *Determinants of Human Sexual Behavior*, Springfield, Illinois: Charles C. Thomas.

—— (1964). 'Marital and nonmarital sexual behavior' in Christensen, H.T. (ed.) *Handbook of Marriage and the Family*, Chicago: Rand McNally & Co.

Elkin, H. (1946). 'Aggressive and erotic tendencies in army life', *American Journal of Sociology*, 51, 5, 408–13.

Elliott, M. L. (1985). 'The use of "impotence" and "frigidity": why has "impotence" survived', *Journal of Sex and Marital Therapy*, 11, 1, 51–6.

Ellis, H. (1936). 'The mechanism of detumescence' in *Studies in the Psychology of Sex*, vol. II, New York: Random House.

—— (1939). 'Freud's influence on the changed attitude toward sex', *American Journal of Sociology*, 45, 3, 309–17.

—— (1942). 'Analysis of the sexual impulse' in *Studies in the Psychology of Sex*, vol. 1, New York: Random House.

Engels, F. (1902 [1884]). *The Origin of the Family, Private Property and the State*, trans. by Untermann, E., Chicago: Charles H. Kerr & Co.

Epstein, S. (1994). 'A queer encounter: sociology and the study of sexuality', *Sociological Theory*, 12, 2, 188–202.

Evans, M. D. and Zilbergeld, B. (1983). 'Evaluating sex therapy: a reply to Kolodny', *The Journal of Sex Research*, 19, 302–6.

Everaerd, W. (2001). 'Sex therapy, clinical psychology of', in Smelser, N. J. and Baltes, P. B. (eds.) *International Encyclopedia of the Social & Behavioral Sciences*, vol. 21, Oxford: Elsevier.

Exner, M. J. (1915). *Problems and Principles of Sex Education: A study of 948 college men*, New York: Association Press.

Farber, L. H. (1968). "I'm sorry, dear"', in Brecher, R. and Brecher, E. (eds.) *An Analysis of Human Sexual Response*, London: Panther.

Faulk, M. (1973). '"Frigidity": a critical review', *Archives of Sexual Behavior*, 2, 3, 257–66.

Flew, A. (ed.) (1984). *A Dictionary of Philosophy*, London: Pan.

Ford, C. S. and Beach, F. A. (1952). *Patterns of Sexual Behaviour*, London: Eyre & Spottiswoode.

Foucault, M. (1981). *The History of Sexuality: An introduction*, Harmondsworth: Penguin.

Francoeur, R. T., Cornog, M., Perper, T., and Scherzer, N. A. (eds.) (1995). *The Complete Dictionary of Sexology*, New York: Continuum.

Frank, E., Anderson, C. and Rubinstein, D. (1978). 'Frequency of sexual dysfunction in "normal" couples', *New England Journal of Medicine*, 299, 3, 111–15.

Freud, S. (1977a [1905]). 'Three essays on the theory of sexuality' in *The Pelican Freud Library Volume 7 On Sexuality*, Harmondsworth: Penguin.

—— (1977b [1908]). 'On the sexual theories of children' in *The Pelican Freud Library Volume 7 On Sexuality*, Harmondsworth: Penguin.

—— (1977c [1912]). 'On the universal tendency to debasement in the sphere of love' in *The Pelican Freud Library Volume 7 On Sexuality*, Harmondsworth: Penguin.

—— (1977d [1931]). 'Female sexuality' in *The Pelican Freud Library Volume 7 On Sexuality*, Harmondsworth: Penguin.

Fuss, D. (1989). *Essentially Speaking: Feminism, nature and difference*, New York: Routledge.

Gagnon, J. H. (1975). 'Sex research and social change', *Archives of Sexual Behavior*, 4, 2, 111–41.

—— (1977). *Human Sexuality*, Glenview, Illinois: Scott, Foresman & Co.

—— (1983). 'Modern sexual theory and sexual reform: emergence, transformation, and criticism' in Davis, C.M. (ed.) *Challenges in Sexual Science*, Iowa, Society for the Scientific Study of Sex.

Gagnon, J. H. and Parker, R. G. (1995). 'Conceiving sexuality' in Parker, R. G. and Gagnon, J. H. (eds.) *Conceiving Sexuality: Approaches to sex research in a postmodern world*, New York: Routledge.

Gagnon, J. H. and Simon, W. (1973). *Sexual Conduct: The social sources of human sexuality*, Chicago: Aldine.

Gamson, J. and Moon, D. (2004). 'The sociology of sexualities: queer and beyond', *Annual Review of Sociology*, 30, 47–64.

Gardetto, D. C. (1992). *Engendered Sensations: Social construction of the clitoris and female orgasm, 1650–1975*, unpublished PhD thesis, University of California, Davis.

Gebhard, P. H. (1968). 'Human sex behavior research' in Diamond, M. (ed.) *Perspectives In Reproduction and Sexual Behavior*, Bloomington: Indiana University Press.

—— (1976). 'The Institute' in Weinberg, M. S. (ed.) *Sex Research: Studies from the Kinsey Institute*, New York: Oxford University Press.

Geer, J. H. and O'Donohue, W. T. (eds.) (1987). *Theories of Human Sexuality*, New York: Plenum Press.

Gergen, K. J. (1985). 'The social constructionist movement in modern psychology', *American Psychologist*, 40, 3, 266–75.

Giddens, A. (1989). *Sociology*, Cambridge: Polity Press.

—— (1992). *The Transformation of Intimacy*, Cambridge: Polity Press.

Gochros, H. L. and Schultz, L. G. (eds.) (1972). *Human Sexuality and Social Work*, New York: Association Press.

Goettsch, S. L. (1987). 'Textbook sexual inadequacy? A review of sexuality texts', *Teaching Sociology*, 15, 3, 324–38.

Goodman, N. (1980). 'On starmaking', *Synthese*, 45, 211–15.

Goren, E. (2003). 'America's love affair with technology: the transformation of sexuality and the self over the 20th Century', *Psychoanalytic Psychology*, 20, 3, 487–508.

Gould, S. J. (1991). *Bully for Brontosaurus: Reflections in natural history*, London: Hutchinson Radius.

Gregersen, E. (1994). *The World of Human Sexuality: Behaviors, customs and beliefs*, New York: Irvington.

Guttmacher, A. F. (1970). 'Effective therapy for sexual invalidism: *Human Sexual Inadequacy* by W. H. Masters and V. E. Johnson', Book review, *Family Planning Perspectives*, 2, 4, 47–8.

Haeberle, E. J. (1980). 'Sex - health or sickness?' in Forleo, R. and Pasini, W. (eds.), *Medical Sexology: The Third International Congress*, Littleton, Massachusetts: PSG Publishing Co.

—— (1983). 'The manufacture of gladness: some observations on sex therapy' in Davis, C. M. (ed.) *Challenges in Sexual Science*, Iowa: Society for the Scientific Study of Sex.

Halwani, R. (1998). 'Essentialism, social constructionism, and the history of homosexuality', *Journal of Homosexuality*, 35, 1, 25–51.

Hamilton, G. V. (1986 [1929]). *A Research in Marriage*, New York: Garland Publishing.

Harding, J. (1998). *Sex Acts: Practices of femininity and masculinity*, London: Sage.

Hare, E. H. (1962). 'Masturbatory insanity: the history of an idea', *Journal of Mental Science*, 108, 1–25.

Hartman, W. and Fithian, M. (1985). *Any Man Can*, Sydney: Angus & Robertson.

Hawton, K. (1985). *Sex Therapy: A practical guide*, Oxford: Oxford University Press.

—— (1991). 'Sex therapy', *Behavioural Psychotherapy*, 19, 1, 131–6.

Heartfield, J. (1996). 'Marxism and social construction' in Wolton, S. (ed.), *Marxism, Mysticism and Modern Theory*, Basingstoke: Macmillan.

Heidenry, J. (1997). *What Wild Ecstacy: The rise and fall of the sexual revolution*, Melbourne: William Heinemann.

Heiman, J. R., Gladue, B. A., Roberts, C. W., and LoPiccolo, J. (1986). 'Historical and current factors discriminating sexually functional from sexually dysfunctional married couples', *Journal of Marital and Family Therapy*, 12, 2, 163–74.

Heiman, J. R. and Meston, C. M. (1997). 'Empirically validated treatment for sexual dysfunction', *Annual Review of Sex Research*, 8, 148–94.

Henslin, J. M. (ed.) (1971). *Studies in the Sociology of Sex*, New York: Appleton-Century-Crofts.

—— (1978). 'Toward the sociology of sex' in Henslin, J. M. and Sagarin, E. (eds.), *The Sociology of Sex: An introductory reader*, New York: Schocken Books.

Hewitt, J. P. (1998). *The Myth of Self-Esteem: Finding happiness and solving problems in America,* New York: St. Martin's Press.

Hite, S. (1981). *The Hite Report on Male Sexuality*, London: Macdonald.

Hite, S. (1989). *The Hite Report on Female Sexuality*, London: Pandora.

Hogan, D. R. (1978). 'The effectiveness of sex therapy: a review of the literature' in LoPiccolo, J. and LoPiccolo, L. (eds.) *Handbook of Sex Therapy*, New York: Plenum Press.

Huaco, G. A. (1986). 'Ideology and general theory: the case of sociological functionalism', *Comparative Studies in Society and History*, 28, 34–54.

Hulett, Jr., J. E. (1940). 'Social role and personal security in Morman polygamy', *American Journal of Sociology*, 45, 4, 542–53.

Hunter, J. (1963 [1786]). 'Of impotence depending on the mind' in Hunter, R. and Macalpine, I. *Three Hundred Years of Psychiatry 1535–1860*, London: Oxford University Press.

Illich, I. (1976). *Medical Nemesis*, New York: Pantheon.

Irvine, J. M. (1990a). *Disorders of Desire: Sex and gender in modern American sexology*, Philadelphia: Temple University Press.

—— (1990b)..'From difference to sameness: gender ideology in sexual science', *The Journal of Sex Research*, 27, 1, 7–24.

—— (1994). 'A place in the rainbow: theorizing lesbian and gay culture', *Sociological Theory*, 12, 2, 232–48.

—— (1995). *Sexuality Education Across Cultures: Working with differences*, San Francisco: Jossey-Bass.

—— (2005). *Disorders of Desire: Sex and gender in modern American sexology*, 2nd edn, Philadelphia: Temple University Press.

Jackson, M. (1984a). 'Sexology and the universalization of male sexuality (from Ellis to Kinsey, and Masters and Johnson)' in Coveny, L., Jackson, M., Jeffreys, S., Kay, L., and Mahoney, P., *The Sexuality Papers*, London: Hutchinson.

—— (1984b). 'Sex research and the construction of sexuality: a tool of male supremacy?' *Women's Studies International Forum*, 7, 1, 43–51.

Jackson, S. (1993). 'Even sociologists fall in love: an exploration in the sociology of emotions', *Sociology*, 27, 2, 201–20.

Jefferys, M. (1988). 'Health, illness and medicine' in Worsley, P. (ed.) *The New Introducing Sociology*, Harmondsworth: Penguin.

Jeffreys, S. (1990). *Anticlimax: A feminist perspective on the sexual revolution*, London: The Women's Press.

Johnson, A. M., Wadsworth, J., Wellings, K., Field, J., (1994). *Sexual Attitudes and Lifestyles*, Oxford: Blackwell Scientific Publications.

Kanin, E. J. (1957). 'Male aggression in dating-courtship relations', *American Journal of Sociology*, 63, 197–204.

Kanin, E. J. and Howard, D. H. (1958). 'Postmarital consequences of premarital sex adjustments', *American Sociological Review,* 23, 5, 556–62.
Kaplan, H. S. (1977). 'Hypoactive sexual desire', *Journal of Sex and Marital Therapy,* 3, 1, 3–9.
——— (1978). *The New Sex Therapy: Active treatment of sexual dysfunctions,* Harmondsworth: Penguin.
——— (1979). *Disorders of Sexual Desire,* New York: Simon & Schuster.
Kardiner, A., Karush, A. and Ovesey, L. (1966). 'A methodological study of Freudian theory', *International Journal of Psychiatry,* 2, 5, 489–542.
Keat, R. and Urry, J. (1982). *Social Theory as Science,* 2nd edn, London: Routledge & Kegan Paul.
Kern, S. (1975). *Anatomy and Destiny,* Indianapolis: The Bobbs-Merrill Co.
Kessler, S. and McKenna, W. (1978). *Gender: An ethnomethodological approach,* New York: Wiley.
Keystone, M. (1994). 'A feminist approach to couple and sex therapy', *The Canadian Journal of Human Sexuality,* 3, 4, 321–5.
Kinsey, A. C., Pomeroy, W. B., and Martin, C. E. (1948). *Sexual Behavior in the Human Male,* Philadelphia: W. B. Saunders Company.
Kinsey, A. C., Pomeroy, W. B., Martin, C. E., Gebhard, P. H. (1953). *Sexual Behavior in the Human Female,* Philadelphia: W. B. Saunders Company.
Kirkpatrick, C. and Caplow, T. (1945). 'Courtship in a group of Minnesota students', *American Journal of Sociology,* 51, 2, 114–25.
Kirkpatrick, C. and Kanin, E. (1957). 'Male sex aggression on a university campus', *American Sociological Review,* 22, 1, 52–9.
Klein, G. S. (1976). 'Freud's two theories of sexuality', *Psychological Issues,* 9, 4, 14–70.
Koedt, A. (1973). 'The myth of the vaginal orgasm' in Koedt, A., Levine, E., and Rapone, A. (eds.) *Radical Feminism,* New York: New York Times Book Co.
Kolodny, R. C. (1981). 'Evaluating sex therapy: process and outcome at the Masters and Johnson Institute', *The Journal of Sex Research,* 17, 4, 301–18.
——— (2001). 'In memory of William H. Masters', *The Journal of Sex Research,* 38, 3, 274–76.
Komarovsky, M. and Waller, W. (1945). 'Studies of the family', *American Journal of Sociology,* 50, 6, 443–51.
Kon, I. (1993). 'Sexuality and culture' in Kon, I and Riordan, J. (eds.) *Sex and Russian Society,* Bloomington: Indiana University Press.
Krafft-Ebing, R. von (1921 [1886]). *Psychopathia Sexualis: A medico-legal study,* trans. by Chaddock, C. G., Philadelphia: F.A. Davis Co.
Krausz, E. (1969). *Sociology in Britain: A survey of research,* London: B. T. Batsford.
Kuhn, T. S. (1970). *The Structure of Scientific Revolutions,* 2nd edn, Chicago: University of Chicago Press.
Lakatos, I. (1970). 'Falsification and the methodology of scientific research programmes' in Lakatos, I. and Musgrave, A. (eds.) *Criticism and the Growth of Knowledge,* Cambridge: Cambridge University Press.
Landis, C. et al (1940). *Sex in Development,* New York: Harper & Bros.
Landis, J. T., Poffenberger, T. and Poffenberger, S. (1950). 'The effects of first pregnancy upon the sexual adjustment of 212 couples', *American Sociological Review,* 15, 6, 766–72.
Lasch, C., (1980). *The Culture of Narcissism: American life in an age of diminishing expectations,* London: Abacus.
Laumann, E. O. and Gagnon., J. H. (1995). 'A sociological perspective on sexual action' in Parker, R. G. and Gagnon, J. H. (eds.) *Conceiving Sexuality: Approaches to sex research in a postmodern world,* New York: Routledge.

Laumann, E. O., Gagnon, J. H., Michael, R. T., and Michaels, S. (1994). *The Social Organization of Sexuality: Sexual practices in the United States*, Chicago: University of Chicago Press.

Laumann, E. O., Michael, R. T. and Gagnon, J. H. (1994).'A political history of the National Sex Survey of Adults', *Family Planning Perspectives*, 26, 1, 34–8.

Lavender, A. D. (1985).'Societal influences on sexual dysfunctions: the clinical sociologist as sex educator', *Clinical Sociology Review*, 3, 129–42.

Laws, J. L. and Schwartz, P. (1977). *Sexual Scripts: The social construction of female sexuality*, Hinsdale, Illinois: The Dryden Press.

Lawson, T. (1997). *Economics and Reality*, London: Routledge.

Lazarus, A. A. (1989). 'Dyspareunia: a multimodal psychotherapeutic perspective' in Leiblum, S. R., and Rosen, R. C. (eds.) *Principles and Practice of Sex Therapy*, 2nd edn, New York: Guilford Press.

Lehrman, N. (ed.) (1976). *Masters and Johnson Explained*, New York: Playboy Paperbacks.

Leiblum, S. R. and Pervin, L. A. (1980). 'Introduction: the development of sex therapy from a sociocultural perspective' in Leiblum, S. R. and Pervin, L. A. (eds.) *Principles and Practice of Sex Therapy*, London: Tavistock.

Letourneau, C. (1881). *Sociology Based Upon Ethnography*, trans. by Trollope, H. M. London: Chapman & Hall.

Levine, S. B. (1984). 'An essay on the nature of sexual desire', *Journal of Sex & Marital Therapy*, 10, 2, 83–96.

—— (1987). 'More on the nature of sexual desire', *Journal of Sex & Marital Therapy*, 13, 1, 35–44.

Levins, H. (1997). 'Sex in 3D; Virginia Masters Johnson's center focuses on dysfunction, disorder and dissatisfaction', *St. Louis Post-Dispatch*, 2 December, accessed online via Factiva database 25 July, 2006.

Lief, H. I. (1977). 'Inhibited sexual desire', *Medical Aspects of Human Sexuality*, 7, 94–5.

Llewellyn-Jones, D. (1986). *Everywoman: A gynaecological guide for life*, 4th edn, London: Faber & Faber.

Llewellyn-Jones, D. (1987). *Everyman*, 2nd edn, Oxford: Oxford University Press.

Locke, H. J. (1968 [1951]). *Predicting Adjustment in Marriage*, New York: Greenwood Press.

LoPiccolo, J. (1983). 'Challenges to sex therapy' in Davis, C. M. (ed.) *Challenges in Sexual Science*, Iowa: Society for the Scientific Study of Sex.

—— (1992). 'Postmodern sex therapy for erectile failure' in Rosen, R. C. and Leiblum, S. R. (eds.) *Erectile Disorders: Assessment and treatment*, New York: Guilford.

—— (1994). 'The evolution of sex therapy', *Sexual and Marital Therapy*, 9, 1, 5–7.

LoPiccolo, J. and Heiman, J. (1977). 'Cultural values and the therapeutic definition of sexual function and dysfunction', *Journal of Social Issues*, 33, 2, 166–83.

McIntosh, M. (1987). 'Sex, gender and the family' in Worsley, P. (ed.) *The New Introducing Sociology*, 3rd edn, London: Penguin.

McIntosh, M. (1992 [1968]). 'The homosexual role' in Stein, E. (ed.) *Forms of Desire: Sexual orientation and the social constructionist controversy*, New York: Routledge.

McKinney, K. (1986). 'The sociological approach to human sexuality' in Byrne, D. and Kelley, K. (eds.) *Alternative Approaches to the Study of Sexual Behavior*, Hillsdale, New Jersey: Lawrence Erlbaum Associates.

Mackinnon, C. A. (1987). *Feminism Unmodified: Discourses on life and law*, Cambridge, Massachusetts: Harvard University Press.

190   References

McLaren, A. (1999). *Twentieth Century Sexuality: A history*, Oxford: Blackwell.

Mahoney, E. R. (1983). *Human Sexuality*, New York: McGraw-Hill.

Margolis, J. (1987). 'Concepts of disease and sexuality' in Shelp, E. E. (ed.) *Sexuality and Medicine*, vol. 1, Dordrecht: D. Reidel.

Marshall, G. (ed.) (1994). *The Concise Oxford Dictionary of Sociology*, Oxford: Oxford University Press.

Marshall, G. (ed.) (1998). *A Dictionary of Sociology*, 2nd edn, Oxford: Oxford University Press.

Martin, J. R. (1994). 'Methodological essentialism, false difference, and other dangerous traps', *Signs*, 19, 3, 630–57.

Martinson, F. M. (1973). *Infant and Child Sexuality: A sociological perspective*, Privately Published, Copies available from the Book Mark GAC St. Peter, Minn. 56082.

Marx, K. (1956 [1932]). *Economic and Philosophical Manuscripts of 1844*, trans. by Milligan, M., Moscow: Foreign Languages Publishing House.

Marx, K. and Engels, F. (1947 [1932]). *The German Ideology*, Parts 1 and 3, Pascal, R. (ed.) New York: International Publishers.

—— (1956 [1845]). *The Holy Family or Critique of Critical Critique*, trans. by Dixon, R., Moscow: Foreign Languages Publishing House.

—— (1967 [1848]). *The Communist Manifesto*, trans. by Moore, S., Harmondsworth: Penguin.

Masters, W. H. and Johnson, V. E. (1963). 'The clitoris: an anatomic baseline for behavioral investigation' in Winokur, G. (ed.) *Determinants of Human Sexual Behavior*, Springfield, Illinois: Charles C. Thomas.

—— (1965a). 'The sexual response cycles of the human male and female: comparative anatomy and physiology' in Beach, F.A. (ed.) *Sex and Behavior*, New York: John Wiley & Sons.

—— (1965b). 'The sexual response cycle of the human female: 1. Gross anatomic considerations' in Money, J. (ed.) *Sex Research: New developments*, New York: Holt, Reinhart & Winston.

—— (1965c). 'The sexual response cycle of the human female: 2. The clitoris: anatomic and clinical considerations' in Money, J. (ed.) *Sex Research: New developments*, New York: Holt, Rinehart & Winston.

—— (1966). *Human Sexual Response*, Boston: Little Brown & Co.

—— (1970). *Human Sexual Inadequacy*, Boston: Little Brown & Co.

—— (1976). 'Sex and religion' in Lehrman, N. (ed.) *Masters and Johnson Explained*, New York: Playboy Paperbacks.

—— (1979). *Homosexuality in Perspective*, Boston: Little, Brown & Co.

—— (1980). *The Pleasure Bond: A new look at sexuality and commitment*, Toronto: Bantam Books.

Masters, W. H., Johnson, V. E., and Kolodny, R. C. (1985). *Human Sexuality*, 2nd edn, Boston: Little Brown & Co.

—— (1994). *Heterosexuality*, London: Thorsons.

Matthews, J. J. (1992). 'The "present moment" in sexual politics' in Connell, R. W., and Dowsett, G. W. (eds.) *Rethinking Sex: Social theory and sexuality Research*, Melbourne: Melbourne University Press.

Maurice, W. (2001). 'In memoriam: William H. Masters, MD', *Journal of Sex Education and Therapy*, 26, 1, 2–4.

Mead, G. H. (1962 [1934]). *Mind, Self, and Society*, Chicago: University of Chicago Press.

Michaels, S. and Giami, A. (1999). 'Sexual acts and sexual relationships: asking about sex in surveys', *Public Opinion Quarterly*, 63, 3, 401–20.

Mills, C. W. (1970). *The Sociological Imagination*, Harmondsworth: Penguin.

Mohr, R. D. (1992). *Gay Ideas: Outing and other controversies*, Boston: Beacon Press.

Moll, A. (1912). *The Sexual Life of the Child*, trans. by Paul, E., London: George Allen & Unwin.

Money, J. (1985). *The Destroying Angel: Sex, fitness and food in the legacy of degeneracy theory, Graham Crackers, Kellogg's Corn Flakes and American health history*, Buffalo, New York: Prometheus.

Morrow, R. (1994). 'The sexological construction of sexual dysfunction', *The Australian and New Zealand Journal of Sociology*, 30, 1, 20–35.

—— (1995). 'Sexuality as discourse - beyond Foucault's constructionism', *Australian and New Zealand Journal of Sociology*, 31, 1, 15–31.

—— (1996). 'A critique of Masters' and Johnson's concept and classification of sexual dysfunction', *Revue Sexologique*, 4, 2, 159–80.

—— (2005). 'Sexual dysfunction and sex therapy' in Hawkes, G. and Scott, J. (eds.) *Perspectives in Human Sexuality*, Melbourne: Oxford University Press.

Murdock, G. P. (1949a). *Social Structure*, New York: Macmillan.

—— (1949b). 'The social regulation of sexual behavior' in Hoch, P. H. and Zubin, J. (eds) *Psychosexual Development in Health and Disease*, New York: Grune & Stratton.

Murray, W. (1976). 'Masters and Johnson: their personal story' in Lehrman, N. (ed.) *Masters and Johnson Explained*, New York: Playboy Paperbacks.

Myerson, M. (1986). 'The politics of sexual knowledge: feminism and sexology textbooks', *Frontiers: A Journal of Women's Studies*, 9, 1, 66–71.

Nagel, J. (2000). 'Ethnicity and sexuality', *Annual Review of Sociology*, 26, 107–33.

Nemy, E. (1994). 'Masters and Johnson: sex researchers still collaborate', *New York Times News Service*, 6 June, accessed online via Factiva database 5 May, 2006.

Oakes, G. (1984a). 'Acknowledgements' in Simmel, G., *Georg Simmel: On women, sexuality and love*, trans. by Oakes, G., New Haven, Connecticut: Yale University Press.

—— (1984b). 'The problem of women in Simmel's theory of culture' in Simmel, G., *Georg Simmel: On women, sexuality and love*, trans by Oakes, G., New Haven, Connecticut: Yale University Press.

Oakley, A. (1972). *Sex, Gender and Society*, London: Temple Smith.

O'Connell Davidson, J. and Layder, D. (1994). *Methods, Sex and Madness*, London: Routledge.

Okami, P. and Pendleton, L. (1994). 'Theorizing sexuality: seeds of a transdisciplinary paradigm shift', *Current Anthropology*, 35, 1, 85–91.

Ollman, B. (1971). *Alienation: Marx's conception of man in capitalist society*, London: Cambridge University Press.

—— (1977). 'Marx's vision of communism: a reconstruction', *Critique*, 8, 4–41.

Opler, M. K. (1943). ' Woman's social status and the forms of marriage', *American Journal of Sociology*, 49, 2, 125–46.

Parsons, T. (1937). *The Structure of Social Action*, New York: McGraw-Hill.

—— (1951). *The Social System*, New York: Free Press.

Parsons, T. and Bales, R. F. (1956). *Family: Socialization and interaction process*, London: Routledge & Keegan Paul.

Perper, T. (1985). *Sex Signals: The biology of love*, Philadelphia: ISI Press.

Person, E. S. (1987). 'A psychoanalytic approach' in Geer, J. H. and O'Donohue, W. T. (eds.) *Theories of Human Sexuality*, New York: Plenum Press.

Pertot, S. (1985). *A Commonsense Guide to Sex*, Sydney: Angus & Robertson.

Pfaus, J. G. (1999). 'Revisiting the concept of sexual motivation', *Annual Review of Sex Research*, 10, 120–56.

Pfaus, J. G., Kippin, T. E., and Coria-Avila, G. (2003). 'What can animal models tell us about human sexual response?' *Annual Review of Sex Research*, 14, 1–63.

Pitts, J. R. (1964). 'The structural-functional approach' in Christensen, H. T. (ed.) *Handbook of Marriage and the Family*, Chicago: Rand McNally & Co.

'Playboy Interview: Masters and Johnson', (1976). in Lehrman, N. (ed.) *Masters and Johnson Explained*, New York: Playboy Paperbacks.

Plummer, K. (1975). *Sexual Stigma: An interactionist account*, London: Routledge & Kegan Paul.

—— (1982). 'Symbolic interactionism and sexual conduct: an emergent perspective' in Brake, M. (ed.) *Human Sexual Relations: A reader in human sexuality*, Harmondsworth: Penguin,

—— (1983). 'Sexuality', in Mann, M. (ed.) *The Macmillan Student Encyclopedia of Sociology*, London: Macmillan.

Pojman, L. P. (1995). 'Relativism' in Audi, R. (ed.) *The Cambridge Dictionary of Philosophy*, Cambridge: Cambridge University Press.

Pomeroy, W. B. (1982). *Dr. Kinsey and the Institute for Sex Research*, New Haven, Connecticut: Yale University Press.

Pryde, N. A. (1989). 'Sex therapy in context', *Sexual and Marital Therapy*, 4, 2, 215–27.

Reckless, W. C. (1942). 'The impact of war on crime, delinquency and prostitution', *American Journal of Sociology*, 48, 3, 378–86.

Reinisch, J. M. with Beasley, R. (1991). *The Kinsey Institute New Report on Sex: What you must know to be sexually literate*, London: Penguin.

Reinisch, J. M. and Harter, M. H. (1994). 'Kinsey, Alfred C.' in Bullough, V. L. and Bullough, B. (eds.) *Human Sexuality: An encyclopedia*, New York: Garland Publishing.

Reiss, I. L. (1967). *The Social Context of Premarital Sexual Permissiveness*, New York: Holt, Rinehart & Winston.

—— (1986). 'A sociological journey into sexuality', *Journal of Marriage and the Family*, 48, 233–42.

—— (1990). *An End to Shame: Shaping our next sexual revolution*, Buffalo, New York: Prometheus.

Richardson, D. (2001). 'Sexuality and gender', in Smelser, N. J. and Baltes, P. B. (eds.) *International Encyclopedia of the Social & Behavioral Sciences*, vol. 21, Oxford: Elsevier.

Riemer, S. (1940). 'A research note on incest', *American Journal of Sociology*, 45, 4, 566–75.

Ritzer, G. (1992). *Contemporary Sociological Theory*, 3rd edn, New York: McGraw-Hill.

—— (1996). *Classical Sociological Theory*, 2nd edn, New York: McGraw-Hill.

Roach Anleu, S. L. (1991). *Deviance, Conformity and Control*, Melbourne: Longman Cheshire.

Robbins, M. B. and Jensen, G. D. (1978). 'Multiple orgasm in males', *The Journal of Sex Research*, 14, 1, 21–6.

Robinson, P. (1976). *The Modernization of Sex*, New York: Harper & Row.

Robinson, P. A. (1969). *The Freudian Left*, New York: Harper & Row.

Rosen, I. (1977). 'The psychoanalytic approach to individual therapy' in Money, J. and Musaph, H. (eds.) *Handbook of Sexology*, Amsterdam: Elsevier/North-Holland Biomedical Press.

Rosen, R. C. (1983). 'Clinical issues in the assessment and treatment of impotence: a new look at an old problem', *Behavior Therapist*, 6, 5, 81–5.

—— (1996). 'Erectile dysfunction: the medicalization of male sexuality', *Clinical Psychology Review*, 16, 6, 497–519.

Rosen, R. C. and Leiblum, S. R. (1992). 'Erectile disorders: an overview of historical trends and clinical perspectives' in Rosen, R. C. and Leiblum, S. R. (eds.) *Erectile Disorders: Assessment and treatment*, New York: Guilford.

Rowland, D. L. (1999). 'Issues in the laboratory study of human sexual response: a synthesis for the nontechnical sexologist', *The Journal of Sex Research*, 36, 1, 3–15.

Ruefli, T. (1985). 'Explorations of the improvisational side of sex: charting the future of the sociology of sex', *Archives of Sexual Behavior*, 14, 2, 189–99.

Sagarin, E. (1968). 'Taking stock of studies of sex', *Annals of the American Academy of Political and Social Science*, 376, 1–5.

—— (1971). 'Sex research and sociology: retrospective and prospective' in Henslin, J. M. (ed.) *Studies in the Sociology of Sex*, New York: Appleton-Century-Crofts.

Sayer, A. (1992). *Method in Social Science: A realist approach*, 2nd edn, London: Routledge.

—— (1997). 'Essentialism, social constructionism, and beyond', *The Sociological Review*, 45, 3, 453–87.

Scanzoni, J. and Marsiglio, W. (1992). 'Sexual behavior and marriage' in Borgatta, E. F. and Borgatta, M. L. (eds.) *Encyclopedia of Sociology*, vol. 4, New York: Macmillan.

Schneider, B. E. and Gould, M. (1987). 'Female sexuality: looking back into the future' in Hess, B. B. and Ferree, M. M. (eds.) *Analyzing Gender: A handbook of social science research*, Newbury Park, California: Sage.

Schneider, B. E. and Nardi, P. M. (eds.) (1999). 'John H. Gagnon and William Simon's *Sexual Conduct: The social sources of human sexuality*. A 25th anniversary retrospective by the authors', *Sexualities*, 2, 1, 113–33.

Schover, L. R. and Leiblum, S. R. (1994). 'Commentary: the stagnation of sex therapy', *Journal of Psychology and Human Sexuality*, 6, 3, 5–30.

Schumacher, S. 1977, 'Effectiveness of sex therapy' in Gemme, R. and Wheeler, C. C. (eds.) *Progress in Sexology*, New York: Plenum Press.

Scott, J. and Marshall, G. (eds.) (2005). 'Sex, sociology of' in *A Dictionary of Sociology*, Oxford University Press, Oxford Reference Online, <http://www.oxfordreference.com>.

Segal, L. (1983). 'Sensual uncertainty, or why the clitoris is not enough' in Cartledge, S., and Ryan, J. (eds.) *Sex and Love*, London: The Women's Press.

—— (1994). *Straight Sex: The politics of pleasure*, London: Virago.

Seidler-Feller, D. (1985). 'A feminist critique of sex therapy' in Rosewater, L. B. and Walker, L. E. A. (eds.) *Handbook of Feminist Therapy: Women's issues in psychotherapy*, New York: Springer.

Seidman, S. (1994a). *Contested Knowledge: Social theory in the postmodern era*, Oxford: Blackwell.

—— (1994b). 'Symposium: queer theory/sociology: a dialogue', *Sociological Theory*, 12, 2, 166–77.

Sennett, R. (1977). *The Fall of Public Man*, Cambridge: Cambridge University Press.

Sevely, J. L. (1987). *Eve's Secrets: A new perspective on human sexuality*, London: Bloomsbury.

Sevely, J. L. and Bennett, J. W. (1978). 'Concerning female ejaculation and the female prostate', *The Journal of Sex Research*, 14, 1, 1–20.

'Sex researchers Masters, Johnson granted divorce' (1993). *St. Louis Post-Dispatch*, 19 March, accessed online via Factiva database, 5 May, 2006.

Sherfey, M. J. (1972). *The Nature and Evolution of Female Sexuality*, New York: Random House.

Simmel, G. (1984). *Georg Simmel: On women, sexuality and love*, trans. by Oakes, G., New Haven: Yale University Press.

Simon, W. and Gagnon, J. H. (1986). 'Sexual scripts: permanence and change', *Archives of Sexual Behavior*, 15, 2, 97–120.

Singer, I. (1973). *The Goals of Human Sexuality*, London: Wildwood House.

Soble, A. (1987). 'Philosophy, medicine and healthy sexuality' in Shelp, E. E. (ed.) *Sexuality and Medicine*, vol. 1, Dordrecht: D. Reidel.

Soper, K. (1995). *What is Nature? Culture, Politics and the Non-human*, Oxford: Blackwell.

Spencer, H. (1970 [1855]). *The Principles of Psychology*, Farnborough, Hants., England: Gregg International Publishers.

Sprague, G. A. (1990). 'Chicago sociologists and the social control of urban "illicit" sexuality, 1892–1918' in Perry, M. E. (ed.) *Handbook of Sexology Volume 7, Childhood and Adolescent Sexology*, Amsterdam: Elsevier.

Stanley, L. (1995). *Sex Surveyed: From Mass-Observation's 'Little Kinsey' to the National Survey and the Hite Reports*, London: Taylor & Francis.

—— (1996). 'Mass-Observation's "Little Kinsey" and the British sex survey tradition' in Weeks, J. and Holland, J. (eds.), *Sexual Cultures: Communities, values and intimacy*, London: Macmillan.

—— (2001). 'Mass-Observation's fieldwork methods' in Atkinson, P., Coffey, A., Delamont, S., Lofland, J. and Lofland, L. (eds.), *Handbook of Ethnography*, London: Sage.

Stein, A. (1989). 'Three models of sexuality: drives, identities and practices', *Sociological Theory*, 7, 1, 1–13.

Strong, B. (1993). 'A descriptive dictionary and atlas of sexology. Robert Francoeur, Timothy Perper, and Norman Scherzer', Book Review, *Journal of Marriage and the Family*, 55, 1, 251–2.

Suggs, D. N. and Miracle, A. W. (1993). 'A critical appraisal of sexual studies in anthropology: toward a nomothetic anthropology of sexuality' in Suggs, D. N. and Miracle, A. W. (eds.) *Culture and Human Sexuality: A reader*, Pacific Grove, California: Brooks/Cole.

Suggs, R. C. and Marshall, D. S. (1971). 'Anthropological perspectives on human sexual behavior' in Marshall, D. S. and Suggs, R. C. (eds.) *Human Sexual Behavior: Variations in the ethnographic spectrum*, New York: Basic Books.

Sumner, W. G. (1959 [1906]). *Folkways: A study of the sociological importance of usages, manners, customs, mores and morals*, New York: Dover.

Swingewood, A. (2000). *A Short History of Sociological Thought*, 3rd edn, Basingstoke, Hampshire: Macmillan.

Sydie, R. A. (1994). 'Sex and the sociological fathers', *Canadian Review of Sociology and Anthropology*, 31, 2, 117–38.

Szasz, T. (1981). *Sex: Facts, frauds and follies*, Oxford: Basil Blackwell.

—— (1983). 'Speaking about sex: sexual pathology and sexual therapy as rhetoric' in Davis, C. M. (ed.) *Challenges in Sexual Science*, Iowa: Society for the Scientific Study of Sex.

Szasz, T. S. (1970). *The Manufacture of Madness*, New York: Harper & Row.

—— (1974). *The Myth of Mental Illness*, rev. edn, New York: Harper & Row.

Tannahill, R. (1989). *Sex in History*, London: Cardinal.

Terman, L. M. with Buttenweiser, P., Ferguson, L. W., Johnson, W. B. and Wilson, D. P. (1938). *Psychological Factors in Marital Happiness*, New York: McGraw-Hill.

Thomas, W. I. (1907). *Sex and Society: Studies in the social psychology of sex*, Chicago: University of Chicago Press.

—— (1969 [1923]). *The Unadjusted Girl: With cases and standpoint for behavior analysis*, Montclair, New Jersey: Patterson Smith.

Tiefer, L. (1987). 'Social constructionism and the study of human sexuality' in Shaver, P. and Hendrick, C. (eds.) *Sex and Gender*, Newbury Park, California: Sage.

—— (1988). 'A feminist critique of the sexual dysfunction nomenclature' in Cole, E. and Rothblum, E. D. (eds.) *Women and Sex Therapy*, New York: The Haworth Press.

—— (1991a). 'Commentary on the status of sex research: feminism, sexuality and sexology', *Journal of Psychology and Human Sexuality*, 4, 3, 5–42.

—— (1991b). 'Historical, scientific, clinical and feminist criticisms of "the human sexual response cycle" model', *Annual Review of Sex Research*, 2, 1–23.

—— (1992). 'Critique of the DSM-III-R nosology of sexual dysfunctions', *Psychiatric Medicine*, 10, 2, 227–45.

—— (1995). *Sex is Not a Natural Act and Other Essays*, Boulder, Colorado: Westview Press.

—— (1996). 'The medicalization of sexuality: conceptual, normative and professional issues', *Annual Review of Sex Research*, 7, 252–82.

Tiryakian, E. A. (1990). 'Sexual anomie, social structure, societal change' in Hamilton, P. (ed.) *Emile Durkheim: Critical assessments*, vol. 2, London: Routledge.

Tonnies, F. (1955 [1887]). *Community and Association (Gemeinschaft and Gesellschaft)* trans. by Loomis, C. P., London: Routledge & Kegan Paul.

Trigg, R. (1973). *Reason and Commitment*, Cambridge: Cambridge University Press.

—— (1980). *Reality at Risk*, Sussex: Harvester.

—— (1985). *Understanding Social Science*, Oxford: Basil Blackwell.

—— (1989). *Reality at Risk*, 2nd edn, New York: Harvester Wheatsheaf.

Troiden, R. R. (1987). 'Walking the line: the personal and professional risks of sex education and research', *Teaching Sociology*, 15, 3, 241–49.

Ussher, J. M. and Baker, D. D. (eds.) (1993). *Psychological Perspectives on Sexual Problems: New directions in theory and practice*, London: Routledge.

Vance, C. S. (1989). 'Social construction theory: problems in the history of sexuality' in Altman, D. et al *Homosexuality, Which Homosexuality?* London: GMP.

—— (1991). 'Anthropology rediscovers sexuality: a theoretical comment', *Social Science and Medicine*, 33, 8, 875–84.

Varela, C. R. (2003). 'Biological structure and embodied human agency: the problem of instinctivism', *Journal for the Theory of Social Behaviour*, 33, 1, 95–122.

Wakefield, J. C. (1987). 'Sex bias in the diagnosis of primary orgasmic dysfunction', *American Psychologist*, 42, 5, 464–71.

Ward, L. F. (1903). *Pure Sociology: A treatise on the origin and spontaneous development of society*, London: Macmillan.

Warren, M. A. (1986). 'The social construction of sexuality' in Grieve, N. and Burns, A. (eds.) *Australian Women: New feminist perspectives*, Melbourne: Oxford University Press.

Waterman, C. K., and Chiauzzi, E. J. (1982). 'The role of orgasm in male and female sexual enjoyment', *The Journal of Sex Research*, 18, 2, 146–59.

Weber, M. (1970). *From Max Weber*, trans. by Gerth, H. H. and Mills, C. W. (eds.), London: Routledge & Kegan Paul.

—— (1985 [1904–1905]). *The Protestant Ethic and the Spirit of Capitalism*, trans. by Parsons, T., London: Unwin Paperbacks.

Weeks, J. (1985). *Sexuality and Its Discontents*, London: Routledge & Kegan Paul.

—— (1992). 'The body and sexuality' in Bocock, R. and Thompson, K. (eds.) *Social and Cultural Forms of Modernity*, Cambridge: Polity Press.

Weinberg, T. S. (1994). 'Sociological theories of sexuality' in Bullough, V. L. and Bullough, B. (eds.) *Human Sexuality: An encyclopedia*, New York: Garland Publishing.

Westermarck, E. (1891). *The History of Human Marriage*, New York: Macmillan & Co.

—— (1934). *Three Essays on Sex and Marriage*, London: Macmillan & Co.

—— (1936). *The Future of Marriage in Western Civilisation*, London: Macmillan & Co.

—— (1939). *Christianity and Morals*, London: Kegan Paul, Trench, Trubner & Co.

—— (1970 [1932]). *Ethical Relativity*, Westport, Connecticut: Greenwood Press.

Whyte, W. F. (1943). 'A slum sex code', *American Journal of Sociology*, 49, 1, 24–31.

Wiederman, M. W. (1998). 'The state of theory in sex therapy', *The Journal of Sex Research*, 35, 1, 88–99.

Wilson, G. T. (1982). 'Adult disorders' in Wilson, G. T. and Franks, C. M. (eds.) *Contemporary Behavior Therapy: Conceptual and empirical foundations*, New York: The Guilford Press.

Wilton, T. (2000). *Sexualities in Health and Social Care*, Buckingham: Open University Press.

Wolfe, L. (1978). 'The question of surrogates in sex therapy' in LoPiccolo, J. and LoPiccolo, L. (eds.) *Handbook of Sex Therapy*, New York: Plenum Press.

Wolinsky, J. (1983). 'Masters, Johnson respond to criticism', *Monitor on Psychology*, 14, 7, p. 2.

Wrong, D. (1961). 'The oversocialized conception of man in modern sociology', *American Sociological Review*, 26, 2, 183–93.

Zeitlin, I. M. (1984). *The Social Condition of Humanity: An introduction to sociology*, 2nd edn, New York: Oxford University Press.

Zilbergeld, B. (1983). *The Shrinking of America: Myths of psychological change*, Boston: Little, Brown & Co.

Zilbergeld, B. and Evans, M. (1980). 'The inadequacy of Masters and Johnson', *Psychology Today*, August, 28–43.

Zilbergeld, B. and Kilmann, P. R. (1984). 'The scope and effectiveness of sex therapy', *Psychotherapy* 21, 3, 319–26.

Zingg, R. M. (1940). 'Feral man and extreme cases of isolation', *The American Journal of Psychology*, 53, 4, 487–517.

Zorbaugh, H. W. (1929). *The Gold Coast and the Slum: A sociological study of Chicago's near north side*, Chicago: University of Chicago Press.

Index

Printed in the United States
by Baker & Taylor Publisher Services

Printed in the United States
by Baker & Taylor Publisher Services